I0465831

Multiple Myeloma New Horizon

With Orthodox and Alternative Treatment

Preface

I have written this book so that the patients suffering from multiple myeloma can understand the disease in detail and choose a suitable treatment for them. This book provides detailed information about the clinical symptoms, complications, diagnosis, staging and treatments. In the last 15 years there has been considerable research and progress in the field of clinical studies, etiology, pathology, diagnosis and treatment of multiple myeloma. Even if we do not have the cure of this disease, but still it is one of the highly treatable disease today. Today we have new and effective medicines, which work in a much better way. There are new treatments for bone lesions and fractures. There are new resources for the treatment of its complications. Not long ago, life of a Myeloma patient was miserable, confined to a wheelchair and he barely survived 2-3 years. At present time, Multiple Myeloma patients are surviving 10 years or more and are living comfortable life. The lifestyle of the patient is getting happier and convenient.

In this book, I have written in detail about Orthodox and Alternative Treatment (Budwig Protocol, which is the best alternative treatment and gives authentic success). Patient can carefully select the right treatment for him. This book has up to date information.

Dr. O.P.Verma

Copyright © 2014 by Dr. O.P.Verma

All rights reserved

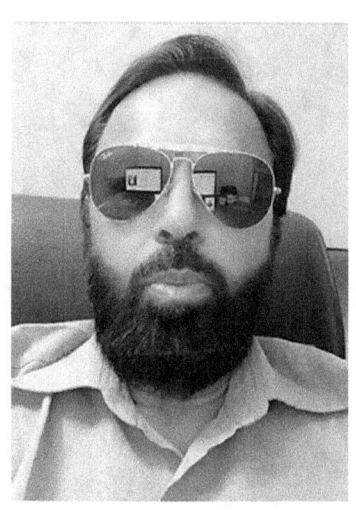

Written by
Dr. O.P.Verma
M.B.B.S., M.R.S.H. (London)
President, Flax Awareness Society
7-B-43, Mahaveer Nagar III, Kota (Raj.)
http://Flaxindia.blogspot.in
http://budwig.in
+919460816360

Table of Content

Multiple myeloma Overview

Multiple myeloma is a painful cancer of plasma cells. Plasma cells are found in the bone marrow and are the main soldiers of our defense system. The Bone marrow is a pulp located inside the long bones. Bone marrow is a factory in our body, where all the blood cells are produced. Remember that this disease was defined as Multiple Myeloma for the first time in 1848.

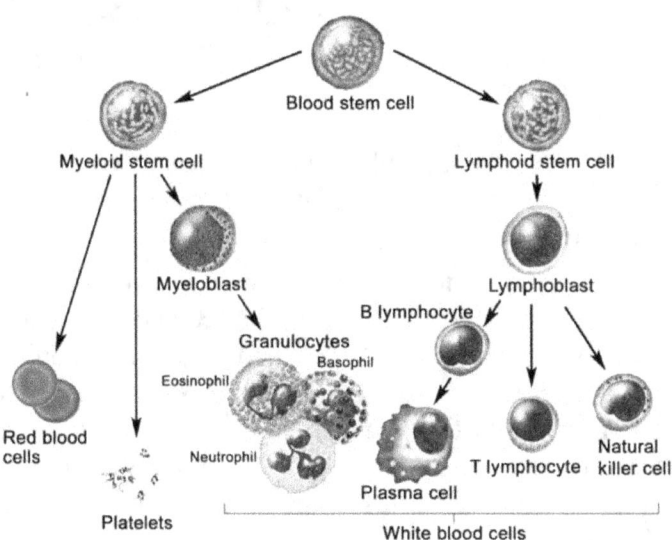

Our body's immune system consists of many types of cells, which jointly fight together with infections and other external invaders. Lymphocytes are the main cells of our defense. These are mainly of two sub types, first T-cells and other B-cells.

When a bacterial invasion occurs in the body, B-cells mature and are transformed into plasma cells. These plasma cells produce antibodies (also called immunoglobulin) on their external surface, which combat with bacteria and wipe them out.

Lymphocytes are found in many parts of the body such as lymph nodes, bone marrow, intestines and blood. But plasma cells normally reside in bone marrow. In addition to plasma cells, normal bone marrow is also the production house for other blood cells such as red cells, white cells, and platelets.

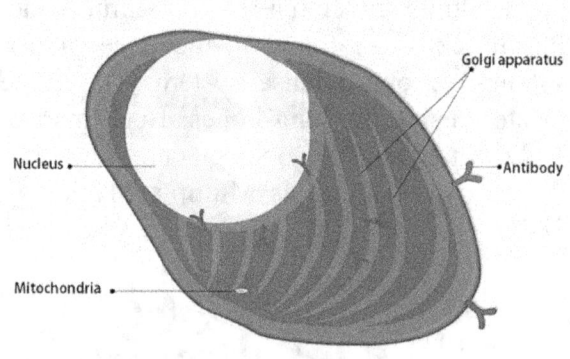

Plasma cell

Golgi apparatus

Nucleus

Antibody

Mitochondria

When plasma cells become cancerous, they grow rapidly and form tumor, which is called plasmacytoma. If the a single tumor is formed then it is called isolated or solitary plasmacytoma, but if more than one tumor is formed then it is called Multiple Myeloma. These tumors are formed mainly in bone marrow.

The rapidly expanding plasma cells in Multiple Myeloma spread in the bone marrow and the other cells do not get enough space to survive and grow. As a result, the population of other cells starts decreasing. If RBC count drops, then the patient develops anemia, suffers from weakness and fatigue, and the body becomes pale. There is a risk of bleeding, when platelets are low (Thrombocytopenia). Infections can occur if W.B.C.count drops (Leucopenia).

Myeloma cells also interfere with cells that help keep bones strong. Bones are constantly being remade to keep them strong. Two types of cells work together to keep the bones healthy and strong. Where osteoblast cells make new bone tissues, osteoclasts break down old bone tissues. Myeloma cells secret osteoclasts activating factor secrete, with the effect of osteoclasts rapidly smelling bones. On the other hand, osteoblasts do not get proper signal to make new bone tissues, consequently the bones become weak and hollow, and the patient feels pain and the bones are easily crack and fracture. With the bones weakening their calcium melts and enters into the blood stream, so that the levels of calcium in the blood begin to rise.

Abnormal and cancerous plasma cells are unable to produce antibodies (immunoglobulins). Therefore they are completely helpless and unable to protect the body. Myeloma cells are similar to many carbon copies of the same plasma cell and they make an abnormal protein (antibody) known by several different names, including monoclonal

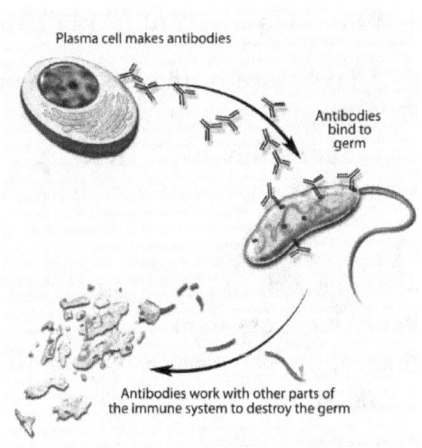

immunoglobulin, monoclonal protein (M-protein), M-spike, or paraprotein. It is the main defect of myeloma. This protein is also called paraprotein or M spike. When the amount of this protein increases in bone marrow and blood, the patient suffers from many problems. Immunoglobulin protein chains are made up of 2 long chains and 2 small chains (light). Many times the kidneys excite this M protein in urine. This protein, which is released in urine, is called a light chain or Bence Jones protein. These can damage the kidneys.

Epidemiology

According to the American Cancer Society, 20,000 new patient registers of Multiple Myeloma are registered every year in the United States alone. Myeloma Incidence is 1% in the US. In African Americans, incidence is 2%. This is the disease of old age; its average age of incidence is 68-70 years. It is more common in men than in women. The average 5-year life span is around 35%. Young patients are more likely to live longer.

In 2010, 74,000 people worldwide died from multiple myeloma. This is the most common hematology cancer after non-

3

Hodgkin's lymphoma. 1% of the world's cancer patients are of multiple myeloma and 2% of those who die of cancer are from the myeloma.

Cause of Multiple Myeloma

The cause of this disease is unknown in allopathy, but some risk factors related to genetic, environment and business are considered important. Here are a few risk factors that could affect someone's chance of getting multiple myeloma.

Age

The risk of developing multiple myeloma goes up as people get older. Less than 1% of cases are diagnosed in people younger than 35. Most people diagnosed with this cancer are at least 65 years old.

Gender

Men are slightly more likely to develop multiple myeloma than women.

Race

Multiple myeloma is more than twice as common in African Americans as in white Americans. The reason is not known.

Family history

Multiple myeloma seems to run in some families. Someone who has a sibling or parent with myeloma is more likely to get it than someone who does not have this family history. Still, most patients have no affected relatives, so this accounts for only a small number of cases.

Obesity

Being overweight increases a person's risk of developing myeloma.

Having other plasma cell diseases

People with monoclonal gammopathy of undetermined significance (MGUS) or solitary plasmacytoma are at higher risk of developing multiple myeloma than someone who does not have these diseases.

Different forms of myeloma

Monoclonal Gammopathy of Undetermined Significance (MGUS)

In this disease, abnormal plasma cells produce monoclonal proteins, but these patients do not have tumors or lumps, and they do not have any symptoms of multiple myeloma. This abnormal protein is found in the blood and is monoclonal. There is no damage to bones, calcium levels are normal, little or no protein is present in the urine, the kidney's function normally and there is no anemia.

Parameter	MGUS	Smouldering Myeloma	Multiple Myeloma
Monoclonal Proteins	< 3 g	>3 g	>3 g
Bone marrow Plasma cells	< 10%	>10%	> 10%
Treatment	Wait & Watch	Wait & Watch	Chemo & Bone marrow Transplantation
CRAB Symptoms	No	No	HyperCalcemia >2.75 mmol/L Renal insufficiency Anemia (hemoglobin <10 g/dL) Bone lesions (lytic lesions with compression fractures)

The risk of MGUS increases as you get older. About 3% of people age 50 and older and 5% of people aged 70 and older have M protein in their blood. The highest incidence is among adults aged 85 and older.

The patient lives normal life. The condition of the disease is sudden, when the blood test for any other disease leads to more serum protein and then other tests show that this protein is monoclonal protein. Plasma cells grow in MGUS but their number remains less than 10 percent. Some MGUS patients (about 1%) can later be victims of multiple myeloma, lymphoma or amyloidosis.

The condition is usually detected incidentally during a routine check-up or investigations done for other disease, when a blood test shows an increase in the blood protein level. The diagnosis is then confirmed by serum electrophoresis test which identifies the abnormal antibody.

MGUS does not require any active treatment, however monitoring is recommended. Monitoring of MGUS includes regular clinical assessment and follow up measurements of serum protein. The serum protein should be checked after three months and then again at six months to establish a firm diagnosis of MGUS. If the paraprotein has remained stable it may be checked annually thereafter.

Shouldering Myeloma

Smoldering multiple myeloma (SMM), a term coined in 1980 by Professor Emeritus Philip Greipp of the Mayo Clinic, describes an asymptomatic intermediate stage between MGUS and active myeloma. It reflects a higher level of plasma cells in the bone marrow and a higher level of M-protein in the blood than does MGUS. Smoldering multiple myeloma isn't yet cancer. It's pre-cancer. But it may get worse and become multiple myeloma.

Smoldering multiple myeloma causes one of these changes:
1) Levels of monoclonal protein (M protein) in your blood that are 3g/dl or higher, and/or
2) Levels of plasma cells is 10% or higher in your bone marrow
3) Absence of CRAB criteria (CRAB: C = calcium in blood elevated, R = renal failure, A = anemia, B = bone lesions)

But if you have smoldering multiple myeloma, your risk of getting multiple myeloma within 5 years is much higher than if you have MGUS. These patients are not treated, but are kept under strict monitoring.

Solitary plasmacytoma

Plasmacytoma refers to a tumor consisting of abnormal plasma cells that grows within the soft tissue or bony skeleton. It can be present as a discreet solitary mass of abnormal plasma cells, in which case it is termed a "solitary" plasmacytoma. The prognosis and treatment of solitary plasmacytoma is very different to myeloma.

There are two main types of solitary plasmacytoma:

Solitary bone plasmacytoma (SBP)

Where there is localized build-up of abnormal plasma cells in the bone. Most commonly, these tumors develop in the spinal column but they may also develop in the pelvis, ribs, arms, face, skull, femur (thigh), and sternum (breast bone).Some people with SBP may go on to develop multiple myeloma – around 50-70% over 10 years – so you'll be regularly monitored with blood tests and x-rays and/or MRI scans.

Solitary extramedullary plasmacytoma (SEP)

Where the clump of abnormal plasma cells occurs outside the bone in soft tissue. These plasmacytomas most commonly occur in the head and neck region, particularly in the upper airways (nose, throat and sinuses), but may also be found in the gastrointestinal tract, lymph nodes, bladder, lung or other organs. There is less than a 10% chance of this disease progressing to myeloma.

Solitary plasmacytoma do not have the typical features of myeloma, which include low red blood cell counts, elevated calcium levels in the blood, or reduced kidney function. And although 75% of people with SBP and 25% of people with SEP have an M-protein (abnormal proteins produced by the cancerous plasma cells), they are usually small and disappear following treatment.

Incidence

A solitary plasmacytoma most commonly occurs in middle-aged or elderly people and is very rare under the age of 30. The median age at diagnosis is about a decade younger than that of people with myeloma, 55 to 65 years, compared to a median age of 71 years for patients diagnosed with multiple myeloma.

Solitary bone plasmacytomas are uncommon and make up approximately 5% of all of the plasma cell disorders. Solitary extramedullary plasmacytomas are even less common. Solitary plasmacytomas occur more commonly in men than women.

Symptoms

Solitary bone plasmacytomas may cause bone pain or fractures. Symptoms depend on where the tumor is located.

Diagnosis

A person is diagnosed with a solitary plasmacytoma when: a biopsy reveals a single tumor inside the bone or tissue comprising abnormal plasma cells; x-rays, positron electron tomography (PET scan) or magnetic resonance imaging (MRI) scans show no other lesions in the bone or in the soft tissues; bone marrow biopsy shows no evidence of myeloma; and blood tests show no signs of anemia, high calcium or reduced kidney function due to the M-protein.

Treatment

The treatment used most commonly for both types of plasmacytoma is radiotherapy. This is possible because by definition, "solitary plasmacytomas" are localized. Radiotherapy involves focusing radiation (similar to x-rays) on the plasmacytoma to kill the abnormal cells. The treatment is generally given over several days to reduce side-effects.

Although chemotherapy is generally not used in addition to radiotherapy, there are times when the types of medications used to treat myeloma are considered.

Surgery is rarely necessary but may be required in situations where plasmacytoma involvement of the bone causes skeletal instability and high risk of fracture. In these cases, radiation therapy may be delayed until after surgery.

Radiotherapy generally provides excellent local and often durable control of the plasmacytoma. However, there is a risk that plasmacytomamay recur or progress to myeloma (particularly with SBP). All people with plasmacytoma require life-long follow-up. This generally involves physical examination, blood and urine tests, and x-rays, MRI or PET scans at regular intervals for at least the first five years after treatment has been completed.

Symptoms of Multiple Myeloma

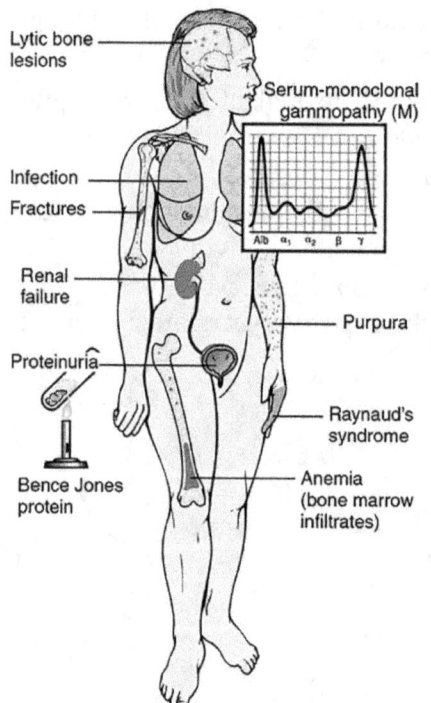

Multiple myeloma is a relatively rare cancer that develops in the bone marrow. Multiple myeloma symptoms may develop slowly over time. Often, early-stage multiple myeloma is asymptomatic (displays no symptoms), and symptoms don't appear until the disease reaches an advanced stage.

The myeloma cells also increase the activity of cells called osteoclasts (which break down bone) and decrease the activity of osteoblasts (which form new bone), causing the bones to dissolve at a faster rate than they are formed. This may damage and weaken the bones, causing pain in the bones (often in the back or ribs), lytic lesions and unexplained bone fracture (usually in the spine).

Its initial symptoms include weakness, fatigue, infections (often pneumococcal), shortness of breath, weight loss, nausea, constipation, increased thirst and urination, increased calcium in the blood, symptoms of pressure on the spinal cord or kidney failure.

As the cancerous plasma cells accumulate in the marrow, they crowd out other healthy blood cells. This may cause several

10

symptoms, such as infection (when WBC count drops), anemia (when RBC count drops), bruising and bleeding (when platelet count   drops). Many times the diagnosis of this disease is made when the patient is assessed and investigated for operation or blood tests are done for other disease. Sometimes a significant difference in the amount of total protein and albumin in blood chemistry produces the suspicion of having a serious disease (note that total serum proteins - albumin = globulin).

The major symptoms of myeloma can be remembered by the CRAB mnemonic. *CRAB means: C = Calcium in the blood elevated, R = Renal failure, A = Anemia, B = Bone lesions*

Bone damage and bone loss

Multiple myeloma leads to bone loss in two ways. First, multiple myeloma cells gather to form masses in the bone marrow that may disrupt the normal structure of the surrounding bone. Second, multiple myeloma cells secrete substances that interfere with the normal process of bone repair and growth.

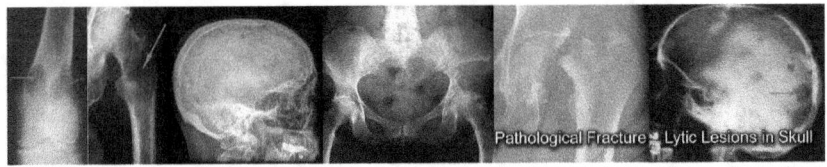
Pathological Fracture   Lytic Lesions in Skull

With weakened bones, people with multiple myeloma often experience bone pain and have an increased risk for fracture. About 93% of multiple myeloma patients get fracture in more than one bone. If there is persistent pain in some place then it is a sign of fracture. The most commonly affected areas are the spine, pelvis, and rib cage.   They are also at risk for spinal cord compression, a medical emergency that requires immediate treatment in order to avoid long-term damage.

Additionally, bone destruction can cause an increased level of calcium in the bloodstream, a condition called hypocalcaemia, which can be a serious problem if not treated immediately.

Common ways to manage bone damage in people with multiple myeloma include supplementation with calcium and vitamin D, exercise, bisphosphonates and other medications, orthopedic interventions, and low-dose radiation therapy.

Pressure on the spinal cord

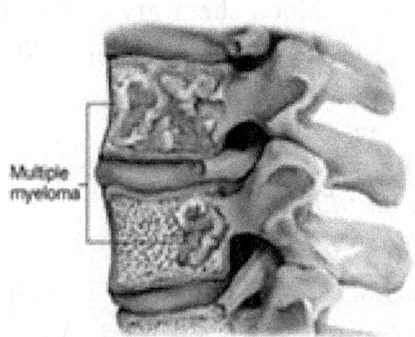

Multiple myeloma

This is a serious disorder, and 20% of myeloma patients may be the victims. Multiple myeloma may cause weakened and/or collapsing bone structures, such as the vertebrae, which may lead to spinal cord compression. Pain, weakness, numbness or tingling may be a sign of pressure on the spinal cord, which may lead to paralysis without immediate medical intervention. Pressure may be at many levels in the spinal cord, so detailed checkup of the spinal cord is very necessary.

Bleeding

Blood clots, nosebleeds, bleeding gums, bruising due to lack of platelets can occur. Occasionally, monoclonal proteins absorb and inactivate the factors necessary for clotting, and can be the cause of bleeding. Hazy vision can be caused by hyperviscosity, which is thickened blood.

Increasing calcium in the blood (Hypercalcemia)

Increasing calcium in the blood may lead to symptoms such as confusion, lethargy, bone pain, constipation, vomiting, frequent urination and excessive thirst. 30% of patients may have a problem. When severe, hypocalcaemia can result in coma or cardiac arrest, so it's very important to identify and treat it quickly.

Infections

Poor immunity and decrease white cell count remains prominent cause of infections. Multiple pneumococcus bacteria is the most aggressive threat, but herpes zoster and haemophilus are also significant. The biggest cause of death in myeloma is considered to be infections. The risk of death in the first 2-3 months of chemo treatment remains the highest.

Hyperviscosity of blood

Increased viscosity of blood can cause symptoms such as uneasiness, infections, fever, headache, insomnia, numbness, bruises in the skin and blurred vision. The condition of the blood is usually four times the concentration of the blood. Sometimes the nose can bleed. The reason for blood thickening is the raised monoclonal proteins level. This can sometimes cause stroke, myocardial ischemia, or infarction.

Neuropathy

Carpal tunnel syndrome, meningitis and peripheral neuropathy are also common symptoms of myeloma.

Anemia

Low hemoglobin may also cause weakness.

Blood clots

People with multiple myeloma are at an increased risk of developing blood clots, as blood clots can be caused by certain multiple myeloma medications. People who are newly diagnosed or who have had blood clots in the past are at particularly high risk. Other risk factors for blood clots include older age, family history, other medical conditions, obesity, and long periods of sitting or lying still.

Your doctor will assess your risk of developing blood clots and may prescribe blood thinners to reduce the risk. Aspirin is recommended to most patients, while low-molecular-weight heparin is prescribed to those at greater risk. In some cases, additional medications may be recommended as well. You can also help prevent blood clots by avoiding long periods of inactivity.

Kidney Failure

In people with multiple myeloma, excess M protein and calcium in the blood overwork the kidneys as they filter blood. As a result, the kidneys may fail to function normally. If the impaired kidney function is so severe that the kidneys are unable to sufficiently do their job of filtering metabolic waste from the blood, it results in a complication called kidney failure. 25% of multiple myeloma patients develop kidney failure.

Medicines such as bisphosphonates etc. also harm the kidneys. If the patient has blood pressure or diabetes, it is also necessary to have a good treatment so that kidneys can be saved from them. Kidney malfunction can be corrected in the early stages.

More than half of people with multiple myeloma will experience a decrease in their kidney (or "renal") function at some point in the course of their disease.

A decrease in the amount of urine is one sign of kidney problems, so let your doctor know if you experience any changes in urination. If your doctor suspects impaired kidney function, he or she will likely perform blood tests to detect certain proteins (such as creatinine) that may indicate reduced kidney function.

Staying well hydrated is one way to manage impaired kidney function. Your doctor may also advise you to avoid anti-inflammatory drugs (such as Advil, Motrin, and Aleve). Depending on the severity of your impaired kidney function, you may undergo plasmapheresis or dialysis.

In myeloma there may be the following disorders.

1- Myeloma Kidney Syndrome

2- with amyloidosis light chains

3- Kidney Stones - Due to Increasing Calcium in the Blood

Clinical checkup

In the eyes, exudative macular detachment, retinal hemorrhage or cotton wool patches can be seen. Due to anemia, the body may look pale. Reduced Platelet count can cause **purpura** or **ecchymosis**.

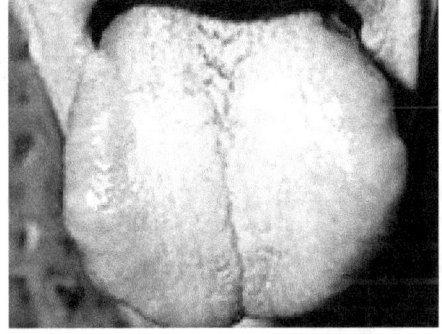

It is normal to have **bone pains** in multiple myeloma. Lytic lesions and pathogenic fractures are common. Liver and Spleen can enlarge in size. Due to protein deposits, the size of the heart may also increase.

Some patients of myeloma may develop **amyloidosis**. They may have the following symptoms.

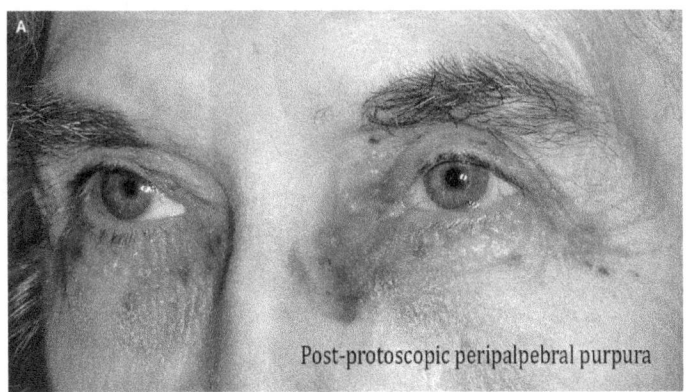

Post-protoscopic peripalpebral purpura

1- Shoulder swelling - With amyloid deposits, both shoulder joints can have hard and rubbery swelling. Carpal tunnel syndrome and skin nodules can also occur.

2- Macroglossia (swollen tongue)

3- Skin disorders - The skin of the lips, ears or fuselage can be on paper and nodules.

4- Post-protoscopic peripalpebral purpura (Post-protoscopic peripalpebral purpura) – If the patient close his/her nose and exhale out forcefully, the dark circles around the eyes are formed. This is a special sign of amyloidosis.

Diagnostic work up

The International Myeloma Workshop developed guidelines for standard investigative work up in patients suspected to have multiple myeloma. These guidelines include the following:

- Serum and urine assessment for monoclonal protein (densitometer tracing and nephelometric quantization; immunofixation for confirmation)
- Serum-free light chain assay (in all patients with newly diagnosed plasma cell disorder)
- Bone marrow aspiration and/or biopsy
- Serum beta-2 microglobulin, albumin, and lactate dehydrogenase measurement
- Standard metaphase cytogenetics
- Fluorescent in situ hybridization
- Skeletal survey
- Magnetic resonance imaging

Consider the risk of acute kidney injury, especially in the setting of contrast medium injection for imaging studies. Take care to limit patients' exposure and maintain hydration.

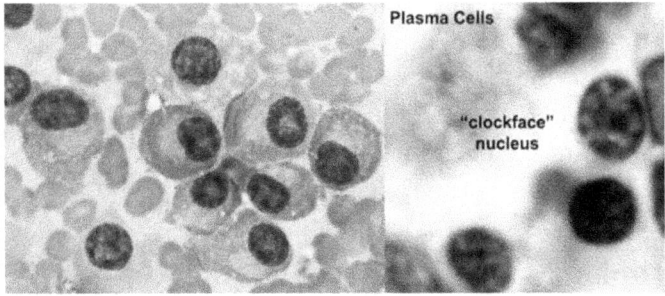

Blood Studies

Perform a complete blood count (CBC) to determine if the patient has anemia (low RBC count), thrombocytopenia (low platelet count), or leucopenia (low white cell count). The CBC and differential counts may show pancytopenia (low blood counts all three types). The reticulocyte count is typically low. Peripheral blood smears may show rouleau formation (raised M proteins in the blood causes the clumping of red blood cells, this clumping of red cells is called rouleau formation).

The erythrocyte sedimentation rate (ESR) is typically increased. Coagulation studies may yield abnormal results.

Biochemistry

- Total protein, albumin, and globulin
- Blood urea nitrogen (BUN) and creatinine
- Uric acid (will be elevated if the patient has high cell turnover or is dehydrated)

Urine Collection

Obtain a 24-hour urine collection for quantification of the Bence Jones protein (i.e., lambda light chains), protein, and creatinine clearance. Quantification of proteinuria is useful for the diagnosis of MM (>1 g of protein in 24 h is a major criterion) and for monitoring the response to therapy. Creatinine clearance can be useful for defining the severity of the patient's renal impairment.

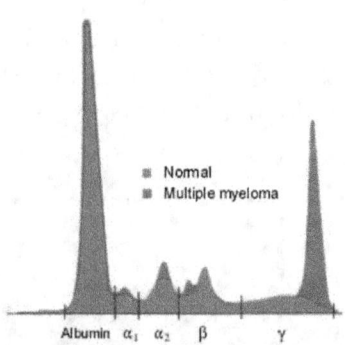

Serum Protein Electrophoresis

Normal
Multiple myeloma

Albumin α_1 α_2 β γ

Electrophoresis and Immunofixation

Serum protein electrophoresis (SPEP) is used to determine the type of each protein present and may indicate a characteristic curve (i.e., where the spike is observed). Urine protein electrophoresis (UPEP) is used to identify the presence of the Bence Jones protein (light chains) in urine. Immunofixation is used to identify the subtype of protein (i.e., IgA lambda).

Chemical screening, including calcium and creatinine SPEP, immunofixation, and immunoglobulin quantization, may show azotemia, hypocalcaemia, an elevated alkaline phosphatase level, and hypoalbuminemia. A high lactate dehydrogenase (LDH) level is predictive of an aggressive lymphoma like course.

SPEP is a useful screening test for detecting M proteins. An M component is usually detected by means of high-resolution SPEP. The kappa-to-lambda ratio has been recommended as a screening tool for detecting M-component abnormalities. An M-component serum concentration of 30 g/L is a minimal diagnostic criterion for MM. In about 25% of patients, M protein cannot be detected by using SPEP.

Routine urinalysis may not indicate the presence of Bence Jones proteinuria. Therefore, a 24-hour urinalysis by means of UPEP or immunoelectrophoresis may be required. UPEP or immunoelectrophoresis can also be used to detect an M component and kappa or lambda light chains. The most important means of detecting MM is electrophoretic measurement of immunoglobulins in both serum and urine.

Quantitative Immunoglobulin Levels (IgG, IgA, IgM)

Suppression of nonmyelomatous immunoglobulin is a minor diagnostic criterion for MM. The level of MM protein (i.e., M protein level), as documented by the immunoglobulin level, can be useful as a marker to assess the response to therapy.

Beta-2 Microglobulin and C - reactive protein

Beta-2 microglobulin is a surrogate marker for the overall body tumor burden. The level of beta-2 microglobulin is increased in patients with renal insufficiency without MM, which is one reason that it is a useful prognosticator in MM. Patients with MM and impaired renal function have a worse prognosis.

C-reactive protein (CRP)

is a surrogate marker of interleukin (IL)-6 activity. IL-6 is often referred to as the plasma cell growth factor. Like beta-2 microglobulin, CRP is useful for prognostication.

Serum Viscosity

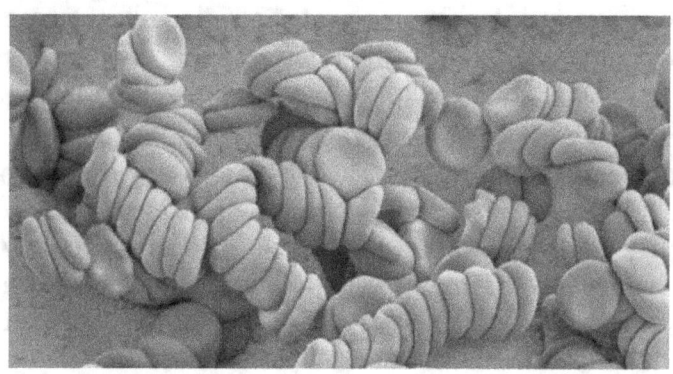

Check the serum viscosity in patients with central nervous system (CNS) symptoms, nose bleeds, or very high M protein levels. These findings may indicate hyperviscosity syndrome.

Radiography

Simple radiography is indicated for the evaluation of skeleton lesions, and a skeletal survey is performed when myeloma is in the differential diagnosis. Plain radiography remains the gold standard imaging procedure for staging newly diagnosed and relapsed myeloma.

Perform a complete skeletal series at diagnosis of MM, including the skull (a very common site of bone lesions in persons with MM), the long bones (to look for impending fractures), and the spine.

Conventional plain radiography can usually depict lytic lesions. Such lesions appear as multiple, rounded, punched-out areas, most often in the skull, vertebral column, ribs, and/or pelvis. Less common but not rare sites of involvement include the long bones. Plain radiographs can be supplemented by computed tomography (CT) scanning to assess cortical involvement and risk of fracture. Diffuse osteopenia may suggest myelomatous involvement before discrete lytic lesions are apparent.

Findings from this evaluation may be used to identify impending pathologic fractures, allowing physicians the opportunity to repair debilities and prevent further morbidity.

Magnetic Resonance Imaging

Magnetic resonance imaging (MRI) is useful in detecting thoracic and lumbar spine lesions, paraspinal involvement, and early cord compression. Findings from MRI of the vertebrae are often positive when plain radiographs are not. MRI can depict as many as 40% of spinal abnormalities in patients with asymptomatic gammopathies in whom radiographic studies are normal. For this reason, evaluate symptomatic patients with MRI to obtain a clear view of the spinal column and to assess the integrity of the spinal cord.

Positron Emission Tomography (PET Scan)

Comparative studies have suggested the possible utility of positron emission tomography (PET) scanning in the evaluation of MM. For example, a comparison study of PET scanning and whole-body MRI in patients with bone marrow biopsy-proven multiple myeloma found that although MRI had higher sensitivity and specificity than PET in the assessment of disease activity, when used in combination and with concordant findings, the 2 modalities had a specificity and positive predictive value of 100%.

These researchers suggest that the combination of modalities may be valuable for assessing the effectiveness of treatment, when aggressive and expensive regimens are used. However, PET scanning has not yet been integrated into standard practice.

Bone Scan

Do not use bone scans to evaluate MM. Cytokines secreted by MM cells suppress osteoblast activity; therefore, typically, no increased uptake is observed. On technetium bone scanning, more than 50% of lesions can be missed.

Aspiration and Biopsy

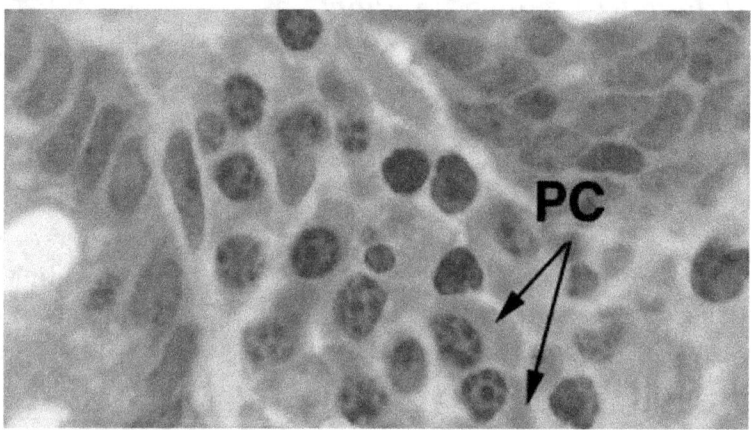

MM is characterized by an increased number of bone marrow plasma cells. Plasma cells show low proliferative activity, as measured by using the labeling index. This index is a reliable parameter for the diagnosis of MM. High values are strongly correlated with progression of the disease.

Obtain bone marrow aspirate and biopsy samples from patients with MM to calculate the percentage of plasma cells in the aspirate (reference range, up to 3%) and to look for sheets or clusters of plasma cells in the biopsy specimen. Bone marrow biopsy enables a more accurate evaluation of malignancies than does bone marrow aspiration.

Microscopic Findings

Plasma cells are 2-3 times larger than typical lymphocytes; they have eccentric nuclei that are smooth (round or oval) in contour with clumped chromatin and have a perinuclear halo or pale zone. The cytoplasm is basophilic.

Many MM cells have characteristic, but not diagnostic, cytoplasmic inclusions, usually containing immunoglobulin. The variants include Mott cells, Russell bodies, grape cells, and morula cells. Bone marrow examination reveals plasma cell infiltration, often in sheets or clumps (see the image below). This infiltration is different from the lymphoplasmacytic infiltration observed in patients with Waldenstrom macroglobulinemia.

Analysis of bone biopsy specimens may reveal plasmacytic, mixed cellular or plasmablastic histologic findings. Approximate median survival by histologic type is as follows:

- Plasmacytic - 39.7 months
- Mixed cellular - 16.1 months
- Plasmablastic - 9.8 months

Cytogenetic Analysis

Cytogenetic analysis of the bone marrow may contribute significant prognostic information in multiple myeloma. The most significant cytogenetic abnormality appears to be deletion of 17p13. This abnormality is associated with shorter survival, more extramedullary disease, and hypocalcaemia. This locus is the site of the TP53 tumor suppressor gene. Chromosome 1 abnormalities and c-myc defects are also significant prognostic factors in multiple myeloma.

Although not as well defined as in other hematologic malignancies, such as acute leukemia, risk-adapted therapy based on cytogenetic abnormalities is at the forefront of myeloma research.

Staging

Staging is a cumulative evaluation of all of the diagnostic information garnered and is a useful tool for stratifying the severity of patients' disease. Currently, two staging systems for multiple myeloma are in use: the Salmon-Durie system, which has been widely used since 1975; and the International Staging System, developed by the International Myeloma Working Group and introduced in 2005.

Salmon-Durie staging system

The Salmon-Durie classification of MM is based on three stages and additional subclassifications.

In stage I, the MM cell mass is less than 0.6×10^{12} cells/m2, and all of the following are present:

- Hemoglobin value >10 g/dL
- Serum calcium value < 12 mg/dL (normal)
- Normal bone structure (scale 0) or only a solitary bone plasmacytoma on radiographs
- Low M-component production rates (IgG value < 5 g/dL, IgA value < 3 g/dL, urine light-chain M component on electrophoresis < 4 g/24 h)

In stage II, the MM cell mass is $0.6\text{-}1.2 \times 10^{12}$ cells/m2 or more. The other values fit neither those of stage I nor those of stage III.

In stage III, the MM cell mass is $>1.2 \times 10^{12}$ cells/m2, and all of the following are present:

- Hemoglobin value < 8.5 g/dL
- Serum calcium value >12 mg/dL
- Advanced lytic bone lesions (scale 3) on radiographs
- High M-component production rates (IgG value greater than 7 g/dL, IgA value greater than 5 g/dL, urine light-

24

chain M component on electrophoresis greater than 12 g/24 h)

- Subclassification A includes relatively normal renal function (serum creatinine value < 2 mg/dL), whereas subclassification B includes abnormal renal function (serum creatininc value > 2 mg/dL)

Median survival is as follows:

- Stage I, >60 months
- Stage II, 41 months
- Stage III, 23 months

Disease in subclassification B has a significantly worse outcome (e.g., 2-12 mo survival in 4 separate series).

International Staging System

The International Staging System of the International Myeloma Working Group is also based on three stages.

Stage I consists of the following:

- Beta-2 microglobulin ≤3.5 g/dL and albumin ≥3.5 g/dL
- CRP ≥4.0 mg/dL
- Plasma cell labeling index < 1%
- Absence of chromosome 13 deletion
- Low serum IL-6 receptor
- Long duration of initial plateau phase

Stage II consists of the following:

- Beta-2 microglobulin level ≥3.5 to < 5.5 g/dL, or
- Beta-2 microglobulin < 3.5 g/dL and albumin < 3.5 g/dL

Stage III consists of the following:

Beta-2 microglobulin of 5.5 g/dL or more
Average survival is as follows:

- Stage I, 62 months
- Stage II, 44 months
- Stage III, 29 months

Treatment

After diagnosis and staging of multiple myeloma treatment planning is outlined. Although it is not possible to cure myeloma today, but it is a highly treatable disease. Because of the field of diagnosis and treatment of this disease in the last 15 years, there has been a lot of research and progress. Today there are better and new medicines, which works in a much better way. There are new treatments for bone lesions and fractures. There are new resources for the treatment of its complications.

The treatment of myeloma is at a unique crossroads, as the work that has been done has created a positive foundation for patient outcomes. We also have the opportunity through our commitment to a new understanding of the disease to get closer in the coming years to our goal of turning this incurable cancer into a chronic, manageable condition.

Not long ago, life of myeloma patients miserable and helpless, he was confined to wheel chair and he barely survived 2-3 years. At the present time, multiple myeloma patients are living 10 years or more while taking cures and are living comfortably. The lifestyle of the patient is getting happy and convenient. Patients should take the right decision regarding treatment to be considered. Second Opinion can also be taken from another oncologist. The following remedies are given for today's myeloma.

Chemotherapy and other medicines

1) **Bisphonates**
2) **Stem Cell Transplant**
3) **Radiation**
4) **Surgery**
5) **Biological Therapy**
6) **Plasmapheresis**

Initial treatment

The initial treatment of multiple myelomas depends on the age of the patient and the severity and presence of complications. High Doses Chemotherapy and Autologus Stem cell Transplantation, among the Patients under 65, is the preferred treatment by the oncologist. The induction chemotherapy is given before the stem cell transplant. In this, the popular regiments used are thalidomide-dexamethazone, bortezomib or lenolinamide-dexamethazone. After giving chemotherapy, in autologous stem cell transplantation (ASCT), the patient's own extracted stem cells are infused into the blood. Nowadays it is considered to be very effective and popular treatment. But there are many risks in it and 5-10% of patients die during treatment. Some patients benefit from this treatment, they can be in 100% remission and their lifespan increases. In the remission period, the disease stays under control, does not increase and for some time patient life in comforts.

Patients who are older than 65 or who have had many complications, usually do not tolerate the stem cells transplantation. Such patients are normally treated and chemotherapy (Melphalan and prednisolone) is given. New drugs like Bortezomib are giving good results. Bortezomib, melphalan and 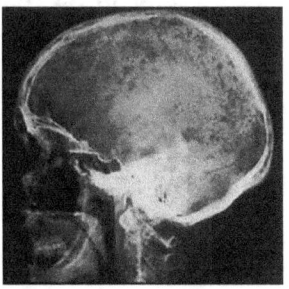 prednisolone or lenalinomide and dexamethasone or melphalan, prednisolone and lenalinomide are giving good results.

Maintenance Therapy & Relapses

Several times after the initial treatment, thalidomide, lenalinomide or bortezomib is given in the form of maintenance therapy. Cancer is a disease that comes back after some time. In such condition, the same treatment is given again or melphalan, cyclophosphamide, thalidomide is given. Dexamethazone is given alone or in combinations. The option of the second stem cell transplant is also kept open.

Chemotherapy

In this, the cancer cells are given to kill cancer cells. But they also cause great harm to our healthy cells and their side effects are also troublesome. Often these medicines are given in combinations and then they are more effective. They are often given with steroids or immunomodulatory medicines.

Traditional chemotherapy drugs

The following medicines are being used in multiple myeloma now a days.

- **Melphalan**
- **Vincristine (Oncovin)**
- **Cyclophosphamide**
- **Itoposide (VP-16)**
- **Doxorubycin (Adriamycin)**
- **Liposomal Doxorubicin (Doxil)**
- **Bendamustine (Treanda)**

Side effects of Chemo

Most side effects of these medicines last for a few days or weeks and subside gradually. Your doctor keeps a watch at the side effects and tells you what medication or other remedies should be used to stop them. Some medicines can cause permanent damage to vital organs such as heart or kidney. In such circumstances, the medicine is immediately stopped and another drug is given a try. The side effects of chemo are as follows.

1- hair loss
2- 2- Ulcers in the mouth
3- 3- Poor appetite
4- 4- Nausea or vomiting
5- 5- Low blood cell counts

6- Weak immunity and Infection (Low white cell count)

7- Bleeding (Low platelet count)

8- Weakness and fatigue (Low red cell cunt)

Chemotherapy Protocols of Multiple Myeloma

Primary therapy (transplant candidates)

- Bortezomib (Velcade)/cyclophosphamide/dexamethasone VCD
- Bortezomib/dexamethasone
- Doxorubicin/Bortezomib/dexamethasone DVD
- Bortezomib/Lenalinomide (Reclaimed)/dexamethasone
- Bortezomib/thalidomide/dexamethasone
- Lenalinomide/dexamethasone

Primary treatment (non-transplant candidates)

- Bortezomib/ Melphalan/Prednisone (VMP)
- Melphalan/ prednisone/thalidomide (MPT)
- Lenalinomide/dexamethasone
- Bortezomib/dexamethasone
- Melphalan/ prednisone (MP)
- Lenalinomide/ Melphalan and Dexamethasone

Treatment recommendations for maintenance therapy

- Lenalinomide
- Thalidomide

Treatment recommendations for salvage therapy

- Lenalinomide/Dexamethasone RD
- Pomalidomide
- Lenalinomide or Thalidomide

Corticosteroid

Steroids are very important drug used in myeloma. They are given alone or with other medications. They also benefit from nausea and nausea caused by other medicines. Increasing blood sugar, hunger puffiness of the face and insomnia are main side effects. When given for long periods, they also weaken the immunity, which can lead to severe infections. Most of side effects start to decrease over time. Dexamethasone and prednisolone are commonly used steroids.

Immunomodulatory drugs

We are not yet fully clear how they affect the immune system. Nowadays three drugs are being used in this category.

Thaliomide (Thalomid) –

Thalidomide was given to pregnant women to stop the vomiting, some decades ago. But it was lifted from the market, because the drug unfortunately caused limb deformities in thousands of babies. But later it started to be used for multiple myelomas. Laziness, fatigue, constipation, and neuropathy are the main side effects of Thalidomide. Neuropathy is a serious pain disorder, and sometimes it doesn't respond to medications. Many times, it may cause thrombosis in the lungs, which can cause pulmonary embolism by entering into the lungs.

Lenalinomide (Reclaimed) -

Lenalinomide is similar to thalidomide, but it is proving very good in myeloma. Its main side effects are low platelet and low white cell count. It can cause neuropathy. There is a risk of thrombosis, but not as serious as thalidomide.

Pomalidomide (Pomalyst) –

Pomalidomide is also similar to other Immunomodulatory drugs. Its main side effects are low platelet and low white cell count. The neuropathy caused is mild and the risk of thrombosis is also there.

Proteasome inhibitors -

They disable enzyme complex called Proteasome. This enzyme complex breaks down the proteins that control the cell division. They also have many side effects.

Bortezomib (Velcade)

is the first drug in this category, which has been approved for myeloma. It is particularly beneficial for the treatment of kidney disorders caused by myeloma. It is given once or twice a week by intravenous or subcutaneous injection. Its major side effects include nausea, vomiting, fatigue, diarrhea, constipation, fever, loss of appetite, and low white cell count and platelet count. There is a risk of

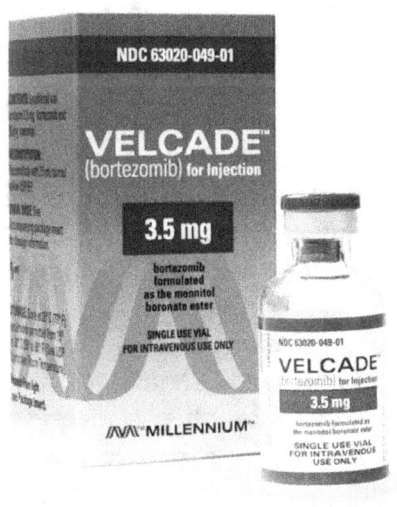

infections and bleeding. Peripheral neuropathy (pain and numbness in fingers and toes). Bortezomib can precipitate Herpes zoster in some patients. To avoid this, acyclovir is given with Bortezomib.

Carfilzomib (Kyprolis)

is the new drug in this category. It has been approved for those patients who have previously taken Bortezomib and immunomodulatory drugs. Its injections are usually given in a 4 week cycle. In order to avoid allergic reactions, in the first cycle, injection of dexamethazone is given before every infusion. Exhaustion, vomiting, diarrhea, breathlessness, fever and low blood counts are the main side effects. It can also cause serious side effects like pneumonia, heart, liver or kidney problems.

Ixazomib (Ninlaro)

A capsule of the Ninlaro is given weakly for 3 weeks per week. Cycle is repeated after a interval of one week rest. Nilnaro is only given when other medicines do not work.

Bisphosphonates

Lytic bone lesions (bone destruction) are present at the time of diagnosis in approximately 60 percent of patients with Myeloma, and almost all patients will have lytic bone lesions at some point in their disease course. While the exact mechanism is unknown, bisphosphonates appear to inhibit bone resorption by suppressing osteoclast activity and keep the bones strong. Pamidronet (Aredia) and zolidronic acid (Zometa) are the main medicines for this category. Their infusion is given intravenously every month. Nowadays they are given for two years. Research done in recent years has shown that Bisphosphonates also benefit greatly those patients who have no bone lesions.

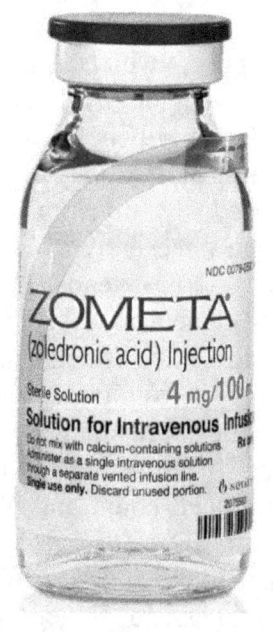

They have a serious side effect **Osteo necrosis of jaw (ONJ).** But this problem is only in 3% of patients taking bisphosphonates. In this, some part of the jaw becomes dead

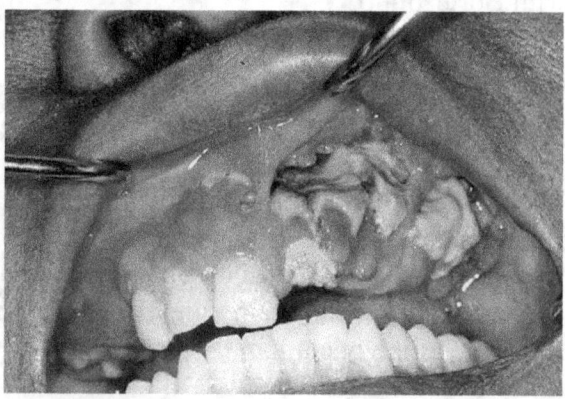

(necrotic), and pain, infection and abscess are developed which don't heal easily. Infections in the jaw and tooth decay is common. The medicine is stopped when it creates ONJ problem.

Stem Cell Transplant for Multiple Myeloma

In a stem cell transplant, the patient gets high-dose chemotherapy to kill the cells in the bone marrow. Then the patient receives new, healthy blood-forming stem cells. When stem cell transplants were first developed, the new stem cells came from bone marrow, and so this was known as a bone marrow transplant. Now, stem cells are more often collected from blood (a peripheral blood stem cell transplant).

Stem cell transplant is commonly used to treat multiple myeloma. Before the transplant, drug treatment is used to reduce the number of myeloma cells in the patient's body.

Stem cell transplants (SCT) can be autologous or allogenic.

Autologous transplants

For an autologous stem cell transplant, the patient's own stem cells are removed from his or her bone marrow or peripheral blood before the transplant. The cells are stored until they are needed for the transplant. Then, the person with myeloma gets treatment such as high-dose chemotherapy, sometimes with radiation, to kill the cancer cells. When this is complete, the stored stem cells are given back to the patient into their blood through a vein.

This type of transplant is a standard treatment for patients with multiple myeloma. Although an autologous transplant can make the myeloma go away for a time (even years), it doesn't cure the cancer, and often the myeloma returns.

Some doctors recommend that patients with multiple myeloma have 2 autologous transplants, 6 to 12 months apart. This approach is called tandem transplant. Studies show that this may help some patients more than a single transplant. The drawback is that it causes more side effects and as a result can be more riskier.

33

Allogeneic transplants

In an allogeneic stem cell transplant, the patient gets blood-forming stem cells from another person – the donor. The best treatment results occur when the donor's cells are closely matched to the patient's cell type and the donor is closely related to the patient, such as a brother or sister. Allogeneic transplants are much riskier than autologous transplants, but they may be better at fighting the cancer. That's because transplanted (donor) cells may actually help destroy myeloma cells. This is called a graft vs. tumor effect. In studies of multiple myeloma patients, those who got allogeneic transplants often did worse in the short term than those who got autologous transplants. At this time, allogeneic transplants are not considered a standard treatment for myeloma, but may be done as a part of a clinical trial.

Side effects

The early side effects from a stem cell transplant (SCT) are similar to those from chemotherapy and radiation, only more severe. 5-10% of patients die during treatment. One of the most serious side effects is low blood counts, which can lead to risks of serious infections and bleeding.

The most serious side effect from allogeneic transplants is graft-versus-host disease (or GVHD). This occurs when the new immune cells (from the donor) see the patient's tissues as foreign and attack them. GVHD can affect any part of the body and can be life threatening.

Drug treatment of Multiple Myeloma

- Melphalan and Prednisone (MP), with or without Thalidomide or Bortezomib
- Thalidomide (or lenalinomide) and Dexamethasone
- Reclaimed (or lenalinomide), Vincristine and Dexamethasone (RVD)
- Reclaimed (or lenalinomide) and Dexamethasone

- Vincristine, Cyclophosphamide, and Dexamethasone (VCD)
- Melphalan, Prednisone and Vincristine (MPV)
- Melphalan, Prednisone and Thalidomide (MPT)
- Vincristine, doxorubicin (Adriamycin), and dexamethasone (called VAD)
- Bortezomib and dexamethasone, with or without doxorubicin or thalidomide
- Liposomal doxorubicin, vincristine, dexamethasone
- Carfilzomib
- Dexamethasone, cyclophosphamide, etoposide, and cisplatin (called DCEP)
- Dexamethasone, thalidomide, cisplatin, doxorubicin, cyclophosphamide, and etoposide (called DT-PACE), with or without bortezomib
- Bisphosphonates - Zolendronic acid (Zometa) and Pamidronate (Aredia)

New medicines in pipeline

Many new medicines are given in patients with relapsed Multiple Myeloma and Relapse Refractive Multiple Myeloma. It is necessary to highlight the following.

Monoclonal antibody

is an element created in the laboratory that acts as an antibody in the body's immune system and eliminates invaders. There are many drugs in this category, such as isatuximab and indatuximab ravtansine. Datatumumabab and Elotuzumab have been approved by the FDA in 2015.

HDAC inhibitors

Lot of research is done recently on HDAC inhibitors. They are given alone or with other medicines. In this category, Panobinostat is approved by the FDA, and ACIL1215 and AC241 are also getting good results. Following regimes are approved by FDA.

1) Lenalinomide and Dexamethazone alone or with Elotuzumab,

2) Lenalinomide and Dexamethazone alone or Ixazomib (Ninlaro), and

3) Lenalinomide and Dexamethazone alone or with Carfilzomib

Two drugs in the proteaezome inhibitors category are also receiving good results of oprozomib and marizomib (NPI-0052), especially the merizomib with pomalidomide.

Certain chemotherapy drugs such as the Evomela and Small Molecular Inhibitors such as Venclexta and selinexor may also prove beneficial.

Treatment of Complications

Anemia

Ricobinant Erythroprotein (40,000 units subcutaneously per week) is given for anemia. In severe cases, peck cell transfusion is given. If iron is lacking then Iron injection is given. From time to time, patient's iron, transferritin and ferritin should be checked.

Hypercalcemia

For this, bisphosphonates are given with diuretics, adequate water, calcitonin or prednisolone.

Hyperunicemia - If too much uric acid, allopurinol can be given.

Kidney failure

Patients with Kidney failure should take adequate water and fluids. If the amount of 24 hours urine remains up to 2 liters, then despite the Bence Jones proteinuria ($\geq$ 10 to 30 g / day), kidney can be saved. We have to do our utmost to save the kidney from the damage. Plasma Exchange gives impressive results in some patients. Dialysis has to be done when chronic kidney failure has developed.

Infection

Many a times Bortezomib causes neutropenia (low white cell count) and herpes zoster infections. These patients are given acyclovir, Valacyclovir or Famciclovir.

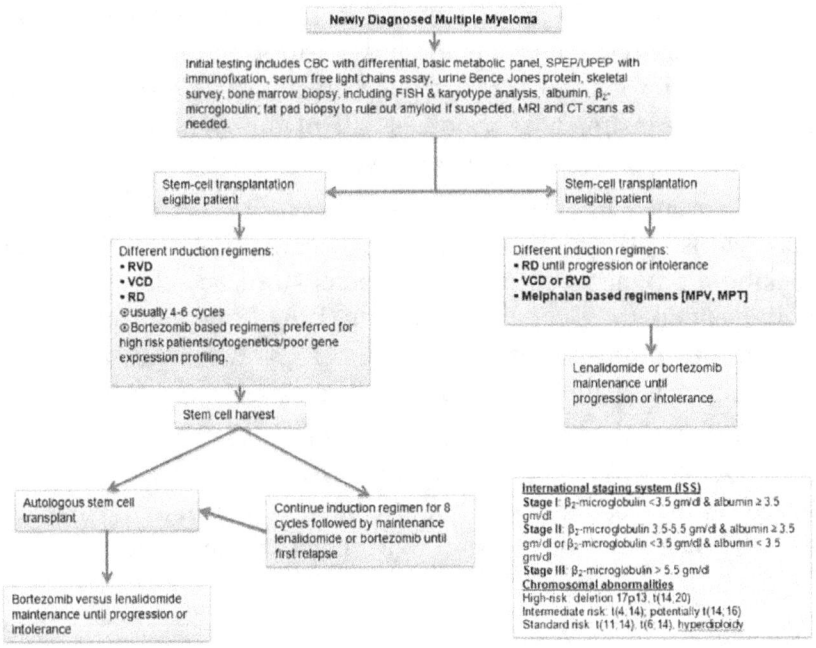

Newly Diagnosed Multiple Myeloma

Initial testing includes CBC with differential, basic metabolic panel, SPEP/UPEP with immunofixation, serum free light chains assay; urine Bence Jones protein; skeletal survey; bone marrow biopsy, including FISH & karyotype analysis, albumin, β₂-microglobulin; fat pad biopsy to rule out amyloid if suspected. MRI and CT scans as needed.

Stem-cell transplantation eligible patient

Stem-cell transplantation ineligible patient

Different induction regimens:
- RVD
- VCD
- RD
@usually 4-6 cycles
@Bortezomib based regimens preferred for high risk patients/cytogenetics/poor gene expression profiling.

Different induction regimens:
- RD until progression or intolerance
- VCD or RVD
- Melphalan based regimens [MPV, MPT]

Lenalidomide or bortezomib maintenance until progression or intolerance.

Stem cell harvest

Autologous stem cell transplant

Continue induction regimen for 8 cycles followed by maintenance lenalidomide or bortezomib until first relapse

International staging system (ISS)
Stage I: β₂-microglobulin <3.5 gm/dl & albumin ≥ 3.5 gm/dl
Stage II: β₂-microglobulin 3.5-5.5 gm/dl & albumin ≥ 3.5 gm/dl or β₂-microglobulin <3.5 gm/dl & albumin < 3.5 gm/dl
Stage III: β₂-microglobulin > 5.5 gm/dl
Chromosomal abnormalities
High-risk: deletion 17p13, t(14,20)
Intermediate risk: t(4,14); potentially t(14;16)
Standard risk: t(11,14), t(6,14), hyperdiploidy

Bortezomib versus lenalidomide maintenance until progression or intolerance

Prognosis and survival for multiple myeloma

If you have multiple myeloma, you may have questions about your prognosis. A prognosis is the doctor's best estimate of how cancer will affect someone and how it will respond to treatment. Prognosis and survival depend on many factors. Only a doctor familiar with your medical history, the type, stage and characteristics of your cancer, the treatments chosen and the response to treatment can process all of this data together with survival statistics to arrive at a prognosis.

A prognostic factor is an aspect of the cancer or a characteristic of the person that the doctor will consider when making a prognosis. A predictive factor influences how a cancer will respond to a certain treatment. Prognostic and predictive factors are often discussed together. They both play a part in deciding on a treatment plan and a prognosis.

Multiple myeloma patients live for 1 to 10 years or more. The average life span is 3 years. Prognosis of this disease is based on the population of tumor cells and their rate of division. The following are prognostic and predictive factors for multiple myeloma.

Stage

People who have a lower stage of multiple myeloma usually have a better prognosis.

Age

Younger people have a better prognosis than older people.

Blood test results

The results of certain blood tests are important in determining the prognosis for people with multiple myeloma.

Beta-2-microglobulin

Beta-2-microglobulin is a protein found on the surface of myeloma cells that plays a role in the immune response. A higher level of beta-2-microglobulin predicts a poor prognosis. The level of this protein goes up if:

the number of myeloma cells goes up

there is kidney damage

Albumin

Albumin is the main protein in plasma that helps to maintain blood volume. A higher level of albumin predicts a better prognosis.

Lactate dehydrogenase

Lactate dehydrogenase (LD) is used to help understand how much cancer is in the body (called tumor burden). A higher level of LD predicts a poorer prognosis.

Creatinine

Creatinine is a waste product of muscle breakdown that is removed from the blood by the kidneys. Measuring the creatinine level shows how well the kidneys are working. People with multiple myeloma who have a high creatinine level have a poorer prognosis. Dialysis can help improve kidney function in people with multiple myeloma.

Chromosome changes

Doctors look at cells removed from the bone marrow to see if there are changes to the chromosomes. Some changes to chromosomes are linked to a poorer prognosis, including:

1) A missing chromosome 13 (called a deletion)
2) Missing part of chromosome 17 (called a 17p deletion)
3) A rearranged chromosome 14 (called a translocation)

4) An extra copy of part of chromosome 1 (called a gain or amplification)

Risk stratification based on chromosome changes

Doctors can predict which people with multiple myeloma are most likely to have the best or worst outcome based on the number and type of chromosomal changes. This is called risk stratification. People will be told if they are good (low) risk, intermediate risk or high risk.

1) Good (low) risk – likely to survive 8 to 10 years
2) Intermediate risk – likely to survive 5 years
3) High risk – likely to survive less than 2 years

Plasma cell labelling index

The plasma cell labelling index (PCLI) measures how fast myeloma cells are growing in a sample of cells removed from the bone marrow. A high PCLI predicts that the myeloma cells are growing quickly and is linked to a poor prognosis.

Performance status

Performance status is ranked on a scale of 0 to 4. A lower number indicates that a person is in better health and is able to be more active than a person with a higher number. Performance status is important in multiple myeloma because people who have a good performance status are able to withstand intensive treatments that may have a better outcome but have more side effects.

Response to treatment

People whose cancer responds well to treatment and go into complete remission have a better prognosis than people whose cancer does not respond to the initial treatment.

Genetic signatures

Gene expression profiling is a way for doctors to analyze many genes at the same time to see which are turned on and which are turned off. Doctors have found several abnormal gene patterns (called a genetic signature) in people with multiple myeloma. These genetic signatures are helpful in making a prognosis. Some genetic signatures are linked to a better prognosis and better response to treatment while other signatures are associated with a worse prognosis.

Alternative cancer treatments

We are fighting with cancer since the dawn of history. Every year we discover new diagnostic modalities, better radiotherapy techniques and lots of new chemotherapy drugs. But we have completely failed to defeat this disease called cancer. Think again, are we really going on the right path? Does conventional Medicine really targets upon the prime cause of cancer?

It's not that more effective alternative treatments for cancer don't exist – they most certainly do. It's just that the allopathic system isn't at all interested in divulging real cures. This is because their expensive therapies generate billions of dollars for the cancer industry.

Chemotherapy Doesn't Cure Cancer – It Causes It!

Chemotherapy does, in fact, kill cancer cells. But it also kills healthy cells, along with a patient's immune system and, really, anything else that crosses its path. At worst, such treatments kill patients more quickly than if they had chosen not to undergo them at all.

There's no money to be made in prescribing prevention advice like eating fewer chemicals and exercising more. The "bread and butter" of the cancer industry is unleashing the next, latest-and-greatest cancer drug. Not telling you how to avoid cancer in the first place.

Many people with cancer are interested in trying any treatment that may cure them safely, including complementary and alternative cancer treatments. There is growing evidence that these alternative cancer treatments give wonderful results. Here are some alternative cancer treatments that are very safe and effective.

- **Budwig Protocol -** *The best Alternative Treatment effective in all cancers and all stages with documented 90% success*
- Laetrile (Vitamin B-17) Therapy
- Gerson Therapy
- Dr. Simoncini Baking Soda Cancer Treatment
- High-dose vitamin C
- Frankincense Essential Oil Therapy
- Immunotherapy
- Hyperthermia
- Oxygen Therapy and Hyperbaric Chambers

Laetrile (Vitamin B-17) Therapy

Introduction

During 1950, after many years of research, a dedicated biochemist Dr. Ernest T. Krebs Jr., isolated a new vitamin from bitter apricot kernel that he called 'B-17' or 'Laetrile'. He conducted further lab animal and culture experiments to conclude that laetrile would be effective in the treatment of cancer. As the years rolled by, thousands became convinced that Krebs had finally found the treatment for all cancers. He proposed that cancer was caused by a deficiency of Vitamin B 17 (Laetrile, Amygdaline).

To prove that it was not toxic to humans he injected it into his own arm. As he predicted, there were no harmful or distressing side effects. The Laetrile had no harmful effect on normal cells but was deadly to cancer cells. Dr. Ernst Krebs stated that we need at least a minimum of 100 mg of B-17 or around 7 bitter apricot seeds to almost guarantee a cancer free life.

Nitriloside is a beta-cyanophoric glycosides, a large group of water-soluble, sugar-containing compounds found in a number of plants. Amygdalin is one of the most common nitrilosides. Laetrile is a partly man-made molecule and shares only part of the Amygdalin structure. Both Laetrile and Amygdalin have been promoted as "Vitamin B-17".

Laetrile stands for laevo-rotatory mandelonitrile beta-diglucoside. The "laevo" part references a purified form of B-17 that turns polarized light in a left-turning direction. Dr. Krebs, Jr. believed that only the left-rotating Laevo form was effective against cancer. So it's important to check the purity of your Laetrile.

How B-17 works (A tale of two enzymes)

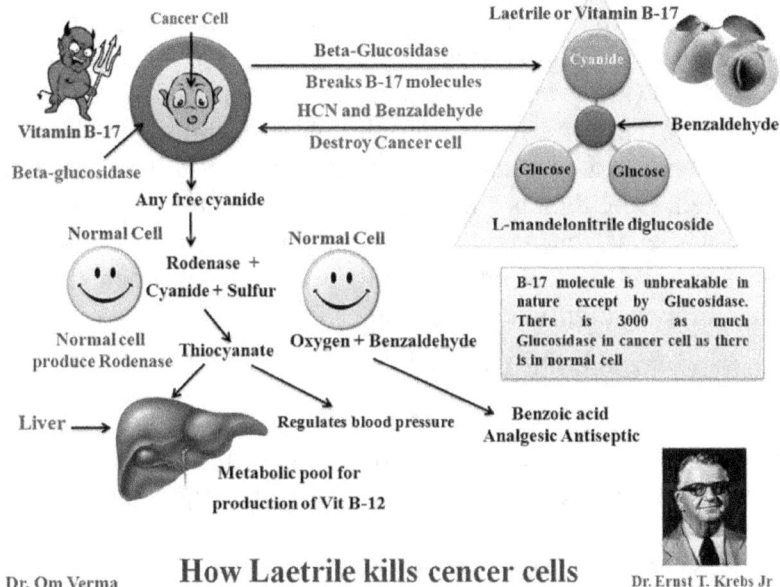

How Laetrile kills cencer cells

Dr. Om Verma   Dr. Ernst T. Krebs Jr

Laetrile, commonly known as Vitamin B-17 or Amygdalin, contains two units of Sugar, one of Benzaldehyde and one of Cyanide, all tightly locked within it. Everyone knows that cyanide can be highly toxic and even fatal if taken in sufficient quantity. However, as it is in locked state is completely inert and absolutely has no effect on living tissue. There is only one substance that can unlock this molecule and release the cyanide. That substance is an enzyme called beta-glucocidase, which we shall call the unlocking enzyme. When B-17 comes in contact with this enzyme, not only the cyanide is released but also Benzaldehyde which is highly toxic by itself. In fact, these two working together are at least 100 times more poisonous to cancer cell than either of them separately. The unlocking enzyme is not found to any dangerous degree anywhere in the body except at the cancer cell where it is present in great quantity. The result is that Vit B-17 is unlocked at the cancer cells becomes poisonous to the cancer cells and only to the cancer cells.

There is another important enzyme called Rodanese, which we shall identify as protecting enzyme. The reason is that it has the ability to neutralize cyanide by converting it instantly into the byproducts (thiocyanate) that actually are beneficial and essential for health. This enzyme is found in great quantities in every part of the body except the cancer cells which consequently is not protected. Here then is a biochemical process that destroys cancer cells while at the same time nourishing and sustaining non-cancerous cells. It is intricate and perfect mechanism of nature that simply couldn't be accidental.

Laetrile - Metabolic Therapy

Metabolic therapy is a non-toxic cancer treatment based on the use of Vitamin B- 17, proteolytic pancreatic enzymes, immuno-stimulants, and vitamin and mineral supplements.

There are three parts to this program:
1. Laetrile
2. Vitamins and enzymes
3. Diet

Phase I Metabolic - Program for the first 21 days

Laetrile

Amygdalin (Laetrile) is available in 500 mg. tablets and in vials (10 cc 3 Gm) for intravenous use. Both forms are used. Two vials of Laetrile are given IV three times weekly for three weeks with at least one day between injections (Mon., Wed., Fri.). Dose of Amygdalin Tablets 500 mg is 2 tab three times a day with meals on the days on which the patients do not receive the intravenous Laetrile. Thiocyanate levels in the blood can be measured during treatment. In general, the patients who do best are those in whom the thiocyanate level is between 1.2 and 2.5 Mg/DL (Philip E.Binzel).

Vitamins and Enzymes

Preven-Ca Caps - Preven-Ca is a comprehensive blend of potent herb and fruit extracts, designed to provide a broad Spectrum of Flavonoids with scientifically demonstrated Antioxidant activity and effectiveness. One capsule with each meal.

Vitamin B15 - One capsule three times a daily at the end of each meal.

Megazyme Forte (Proteolytic Enzymes) Three tablets two hours after each meal (9 daily).

Ester Vitamin C 1000 mg capsule - One capsule with each meal.

Shark Cartilage It has been said that Sharks are the healthiest creature on earth. Sharks are immune to practically every disease known to man. One capsules three times a daily with each meal.

Natural Vitamin E 400 iu - One gel with lunch and one with dinner.

AHCC (Active Hexose Correlated Compound) - Two capsules with each meal.

Multi Vitamin & Mineral Liquid - 1 oz (two tablespoons) once daily with a meal.

Vitamin A & E Emulsion - 5 drops in juice or water three times per day.

Barley Grass Juice - One teaspoon in juice three times per day.

Bitter apricot seeds - No more than 12 every 2 hours 6 times a day.

Dimethyl sulfoxide (DMSO) - DMSO is a by-product of the wood and paper industry. It is known for its ability to permeate living tissue and stimulate cellular processes.

Or Phase 1 Oral

Injectable Amygdalin is replaced with 500mg Amygdalin tablets. Binzel recommends 2 of these tablets with each meal for a total of 6 per day. Otherwise the ORAL Phase 1 includes the same materials as above.

Phase 2 Metabolic - Program for the next 3 months

It comprises the same materials as Phase 1 except that the dosages for the vitamin B-17 as well as the A&E Emulsion Drops change to the following:

Vitamin B-17 500 mg tablets: 1 tablet with each meal and one at bedtime.

Vitamin A & E emulsion drops: 10 drops in juice or water two times per day (suspend for 2 months after 3 months of use).

Diet

Consume those fruits (i.e. seeds), grains and nuts that are rich in laetrile. Consume salads with healthy dressings. For protein patient should consume whole grains including corn, beans, buckwheat, nuts, dried fruits. Real butter in small amounts is permitted. The patients are not permitted anything which contains white flour or white sugar. Take away all meat, all poultry, all fish, all eggs and milk from patients. Margarine is detrimental to good nutrition. No coffee is permitted.

Zinc acts as transport vehicle for laetrile in the body. If patient does not have sufficient zinc, laetrile will not get into the tissues of the body. That's why you should give a spoonful of pumpkin seeds along with bitter apricot kernels. The body will not rebuild any tissue without sufficient quantities of Vitamin C etc.

The Gerson Therapy

The Gerson Therapy is a natural treatment that activates the body's extraordinary ability to heal itself through an organic, plant-based diet, raw juices, coffee enemas and natural supplements.

With its whole-body approach to healing, the Gerson Therapy naturally reactivates your body's magnificent ability to heal itself – with no damaging side effects. This a powerful, natural treatment boosts the body's own immune system to heal cancer, arthritis, heart disease, allergies, and many other degenerative diseases. Dr. Max Gerson developed the Gerson Therapy in the 1930s, initially as a treatment for his own debilitating migraines, and eventually as a treatment for degenerative diseases such as skin tuberculosis, diabetes and, most famously, cancer.

An abundance of nutrients from copious amounts of fresh, organic juices are consumed every day, providing your body with a super-dose of enzymes, minerals and nutrients. These substances then break down diseased tissue in the body, while coffee enemas aid in eliminating toxins from the liver.

Throughout our lives our bodies are being filled with a variety of carcinogens and toxic pollutants. These toxins reach us through the air we breathe, the food we eat, the medicines we take and the water we drink. The Gerson Therapy's intensive detoxification regimen eliminates these toxins from the body, so that true healing can begin.

How the Gerson Therapy Works

The Gerson Therapy regenerates the body to health, supporting each important metabolic requirement by flooding the body with nutrients from about 15- 20 pounds of organically-grown fruits and vegetables daily. Most is used to make fresh raw juice, up to one glass every hour, up to 13 times per day. Raw and cooked solid foods are generously consumed. Oxygenation is usually more than doubled, as oxygen deficiency in the blood contributes to many degenerative diseases. The metabolism is also stimulated through the addition of thyroid, potassium and other supplements, and by avoiding heavy animal fats, excess protein, sodium and other toxins.

Degenerative diseases render the body increasingly unable to excrete waste materials adequately, commonly resulting in liver and kidney failure. The Gerson Therapy uses intensive detoxification to eliminate wastes, regenerate the liver, reactivate the immune system and restore the body's essential defenses – enzyme, mineral and hormone systems. With generous, high-quality nutrition, increased oxygen availability, detoxification, and improved metabolism, the cells – and the body – can regenerate, become healthy and prevent future illness.

Juicing

Fresh-pressed juice from raw foods provides the easiest and most effective way of providing high-quality nutrition. By juicing, patients can take in the nutrients and enzymes from nearly 15 pounds of produce every day, in a manner that is easy to digest and absorb.

Every day, a typical patient on the Gerson Therapy for cancer consumes up to thirteen glasses of fresh, raw carrot-apple and green leaf juices. These juices are prepared hourly from fresh, raw, organic fruits and vegetables, using a two-step juicer or a masticating juicer used with a separate hydraulic press.

The Gerson Therapy Diet

The Gerson Therapy diet is plant-based and entirely organic. The diet is naturally high in vitamins, minerals, enzymes, micro-nutrients, and extremely low in sodium, fats, and proteins. The following is a typical daily diet for a Gerson patient on the full therapy regimen:

- Thirteen glasses of fresh, raw carrot-apple and green-leaf juices prepared hourly from fresh, organic fruits and vegetables.

50

- Three full plant-based meals, freshly prepared from organically grown fruits, vegetables and whole grains. A typical meal will include salad, cooked vegetables, baked potatoes, Hippocrates soup and juice.
- Fresh fruit and vegetables available at all hours for snacking, in addition to the regular diet.

Supplements

All medications used in connection with the Gerson Therapy are classed as biologicals, materials of organic origin that are supplied in therapeutic amounts. The supplements used on the Gerson Therapy include:

- Potassium compound
- Lugol's solution
- Vitamin B-12
- Thyroid hormone
- Pancreatic Enzymes

Detoxification

Coffee enemas are the primary method of detoxification of the tissues and blood on the Gerson Therapy. Coffee enemas accomplish this essential task, assisting the liver in eliminating toxic residues from the body for good. Cancer patients on the Gerson Therapy may take up to 5 coffee enemas per day. The Gerson Therapy also utilizes castor oil to stimulate bile flow and enhance the liver's ability to filter blood.

Simoncini's Baking Soda Cancer Treatment

Dr. Tullio Simoncini is a medical doctor in Italy who has done more than anyone to explore the uses of the baking soda cancer treatment as an alternative cancer treatment. It is known that cancer creates and favors an acid environment and because of this, Dr. Simoncini and others have used sodium bicarbonate as an alkaline therapeutic agent.

The way that acidity seems to protect cancer is not fully understood. It seems that cytotoxic T-cells, which may attack cancer cells under normal conditions, are inactivated in an acid extracellular fluid. Also, the type of acidity that cancer produces, i.e., lactic acid, stimulates vascular endothelial growth factor and angiogenesis. This is like a highway project, which enables a tumor to build the blood vessels that it needs to bring the nutrients for it to survive. So the tumor creates an environment in which it can then exist comfortably.

Baking Soda's Alkalinity Fights Cancer's Acidity

At a pH of about 10, sodium bicarbonate is an antidote to this acidity. It can be used clinically in sterile, intravenous form. This is a liquid, sterile bicarbonate of soda. The baking soda cancer treatment is well-tolerated, even with frequent repeated dosing. Dr. Simonchini also injects soda bicarb solution directly into the tumors at his center.

Cancer a Fungus problem?

Dr. Simonchini says that cancer is caused by fungus However, it is useful to know that not only does sodium bicarbonate disrupt the comfortable environment of tumors, but it also has anti-fungal effect.

Best Alternative Treatment - Budwig Protocol

90% documented success in all types of Cancers

Bonding of Alpha-Linolenic Acid and Sulfurated Protein

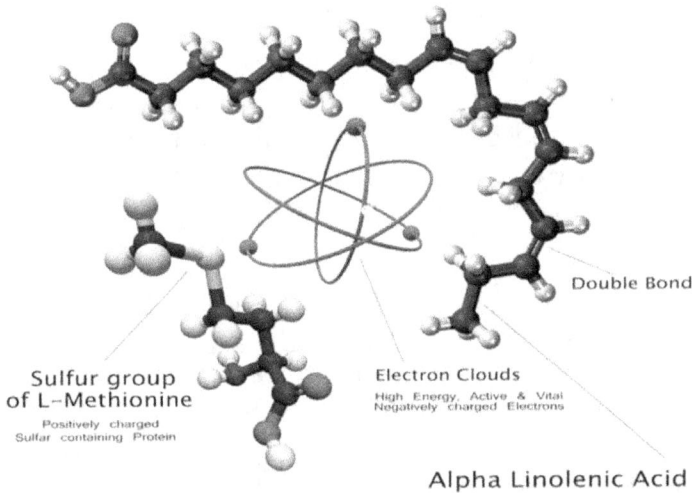

Double Bond

Sulfur group
of L–Methionine
Positively charged
Sulfar containing Protein

Electron Clouds
High Energy, Active & Vital
Negatively charged Electrons

Alpha Linolenic Acid

Dr. Budwig has been referred to as a top European cancer research scientist, biochemist, pharmacologist, and physicist. Dr. Budwig was a seven-time Nobel Prize nominee.

In Germany in 1952, she was the central government's senior expert for fats and pharmaceutical drugs. She's considered one of the world's leading authorities on fats and oils. Her research has shown the tremendous effects that commercially processed fats and oils (having Trans fatty acids) have in destroying cell membranes and lowering the voltage in the cells of our bodies, which then result in chronic and terminal disease including cancer.

What we have forgotten is that we are body electric. The cells of our body fire electrically. They have a nucleus in the center of the cell which is positively charged, and the cell membrane, which is the outer lining of the cell, is negatively charged. We are all aware of how fats clog up our veins and arteries and are the leading cause of heart attacks, but we never looked beyond the end of our noses to see how these very dangerous fats and oils are affecting the overall health of our minds and bodies at the cellular level.

Dr. Budwig discovered that when unsaturated fats have been chemically treated, their unsaturated qualities are destroyed and the field of electrons removed. This commercial processing of fats destroys the field of electrons that the cell membranes (60-75 trillion cells) in our bodies must have to fire properly (i.e. function properly).

The fats' ability to associate with protein and thereby to achieve water solubility in the fluids of the living body is destroyed. As Dr. Budwig put it, "the battery is dead because the electrons in these fats and oils recharge it." When the electrons are destroyed the fats are no longer active and cannot flow into the capillaries and through the fine capillary networks. This is when circulation problems arise.

Without the proper metabolism of fats in our bodies, every vital function and every organ is affected. This includes the generation of new life and new cells. Our bodies produce over 500 million new cells daily. Dr. Budwig points out that in growing new cells, there is a polarity between the electrically positive nucleus and the electrically negative cell membrane with its high unsaturated fatty acids. During cell division, the cell, and new daughter cell must contain enough electron-rich fatty acids in the cell's surface area to divide off completely from the old cell. When this process is interrupted the body begins to die. In essence, these commercially processed fats and oils are shutting down the electrical field of the cells allowing chronic and terminal diseases to take hold of our bodies.

A very good example would be tumors. Dr. Budwig noted that "The formation of tumors usually happens as follows. In those body areas which normally host many growth processes, such as in the skin and membranes, the glandular organs, for example, the liver and pancreas or the glands in the stomach and intestinal tract—it is here that the growth processes are brought to a stand still. Because the polarity is missing, due to the lack of electron rich highly unsaturated fat, the course of growth is disturbed—the surface-active fats are not present; the substance becomes inactive before the maturing and shedding process of the cells ever takes place, which results in the formation of tumors."

She pointed out that this can be reversed by providing the simple foods, cottage cheese, and flax seed oil, which revises the stagnated growth processes. This naturally causes the tumor or tumors present to dissolve and the whole range of symptoms which indicate a "dead battery are cured." Dr. Budwig did not believe in the use of growth-inhibiting treatments such as chemotherapy or radiation. She was quoted as saying "I flat declare that

55

the usual hospital treatments today, in a case of tumorous growth, most certainly leads to worsening of the disease or a speedier death, and in healthy people, quickly causes cancer."

Dr. Budwig discovered that when she combined flaxseed oil, with its powerful healing nature of essential electron rich unsaturated fats, and cottage cheese, which is rich in sulfur protein, the bonding produced makes the oil water soluble and easily absorbed into the cell membrane.

I found testimonials of people from around the world who had been diagnosed with terminal cancer (all types of cancer), sent home to die and were now living healthy, normal lives. Not only had Dr. Budwig been using her protocol for treating cancer in Europe, but she also treated other chronic diseases such as arthritis, heart infarction, irregular heart beat, psoriasis, eczema (other skin diseases), immune deficiency syndromes (Multiple Sclerosis and other autoimmune diseases), diabetes, lungs (respiratory conditions), stomach ulcers, liver, prostate, strokes, brain tumors, brain (strengthens activity), arteriosclerosis and other chronic diseases. Dr. Budwig's protocol proved successful where orthodox traditional medicine was failing.

Prime Cause of Cancer

We are fighting with cancer since the dawn of history. Every year we discover new diagnostic modalities, better radiotherapy techniques and lots of new chemotherapy drugs. But we have completely failed to defeat this disease called cancer. Think again, are we really going on the right path? Does conventional Medicine really targets upon the prime cause of cancer???

Otto Warburg – Biography

Otto Heinrich Warburg (October 8, 1883 – August 1, 1970), son of physicist Emil Warburg, was a German physiologist, medical doctor and Nobel laureate. His mother was the daughter of a Protestant family of bankers and civil servants from Baden. Warburg studied chemistry under the great Emil Fischer, and earned his "Doctor of Chemistry" in Berlin in 1906. He then earned the degree of "Doctor of Medicine" in Heidelberg in 1911. Between 1908 and 1914, Warburg was affiliated with the Naples Marine Biological Station, in Naples, Italy, where he conducted research.

He served as an officer in the elite Uhlan (cavalry regiment) during the First World War, and was given the Iron Cross (1st Class) award for his bravery. Warburg is considered one of the 20th century's leading biochemists. Towards the end of the war, Albert Einstein, who had been a friend of Warburg's father Emil, wrote Warburg asking him to leave the army and return to academia, since it would be a tragedy for the world to lose his talents. Einstein and Warburg later became friends, and Einstein's work in physics had great influence on Otto's biochemical research.

While working at the Marine Biological Station, Warburg performed research on oxygen consumption in sea urchin eggs

57

after fertilization, and proved that upon fertilization, the rate of respiration increases by as much as six fold. His experiments also proved that iron is essential for the development of the larval stage.

In 1918, Warburg was appointed professor at the Kaiser Wilhelm Institute for Biology in Berlin-Dahlem. By 1931 he was promoted as director of the Kaiser Wilhelm Institute for Cell Physiology, which was later on, renamed the Max Planck Society. Warburg investigated the metabolism of tumors and the respiration of cells, particularly cancer cells, and in 1931 was awarded the Nobel Prize in Physiology for his "discovery of the nature and mode of action of the respiratory enzyme."

Nomination for a second Nobel Prize

In 1944, Warburg was nominated for a second Nobel Prize in Physiology by Albert Szent-Györgyi, for his work on nicotinamide, the mechanism and enzymes involved in fermentation, and the discovery of flavin (in yellow enzymes), but was prevented from receiving it by Adolf Hitler's regime.

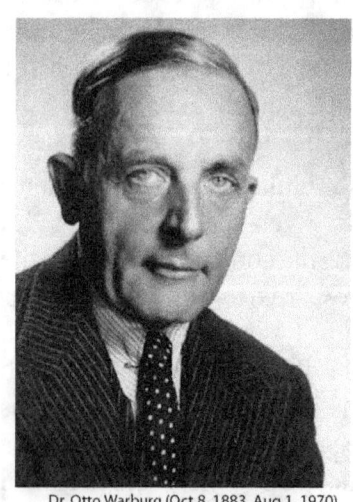

Dr. Otto Warburg (Oct 8, 1883 Aug 1, 1970)

Otto Warburg edited and had much of his original work published in The Metabolism of Tumors and wrote New Methods of Cell Physiology (1962). Otto Warburg was thrilled when Oxford University awarded him an honorary doctorate.

In his later years, Warburg was convinced that illness is resulted from pollution; this caused him to become a bit of a health advocate. He insisted on eating bread made from wheat grown organically on his farm. When he visited restaurants, he often made arrangements to pay the full price for a cup of tea, but to only be served boiling water, from which he would make tea with a tea bag he had brought with him. He was also known to go to significant lengths to obtain organic butter, the quality of which he trusted.

The Otto Warburg Medal

The Otto Warburg Medal is intended to commemorate Warburg's outstanding achievements. It has been awarded by the German Society for Biochemistry and Molecular Biology since 1963. The prize honors and encourages pioneering achievements in fundamental biochemical and molecular biological research. The Otto Warburg Medal is regarded as the highest award for biochemists and molecular biologists in Germany.

Prime cause of Cancer

Warburg hypothesized that cancer growth is caused by tumor cells mainly generating energy (as e.g. adenosine triphosphate / ATP) by anaerobic breakdown of glucose (known as fermentation, or anaerobic respiration). This is in contrast to healthy cells, which mainly generate energy from oxidative breakdown of pyruvate. Pyruvate is an end product of glycolysis, and is oxidized within the mitochondria. Hence, and according to Warburg, cancer should be interpreted as a mitochondrial dysfunction.

In short, Warburg summarized that all normal cells absolutely require oxygen, but cancer cells can live without oxygen - a rule without exception. Deprive a cell 35% of its oxygen for 48 hours and it would become cancerous. **Dr. Otto Warburg clearly mentioned that the root cause of cancer is lack of oxygen in the cells.**

He also discovered that cancer cells are anaerobic (do not breathe oxygen), get the energy by fermenting glucose and produce levo-rotating lactic acid, and the body becomes acidic. Cancer cannot survive in the presence of high levels of oxygen, as found in an alkaline state.

He postulated that sulfur containing protein and some unknown fat is required to attract oxygen into the cell. This fat plays a major role in the respiration and functioning of Warburg respiratory enzyme. He thought it would be butyric acid and made experiment, but this attempt was a failure. For many decades scientists were trying to identify this unknown and mysterious fat but nobody succeeded (Otto Warburg, Wikipedia).

Dr. Johanna Budwig - Biography & Science

Birth of an angel

A lovely couple, Hermann Budwig and Elisabeth, lived in Essen town of Germany situated on the bank of river Ruhr. On the eve of 30th September, 1908 Elisabeth delivered a brilliant and lucky angel. Hermann and 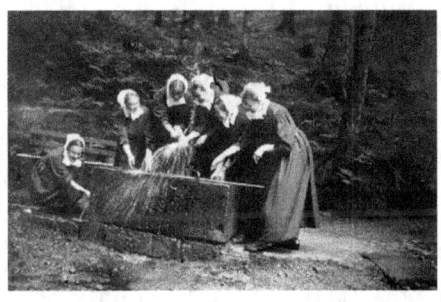 Elisabeth were very happy, and celebrating. They called her Johanna. In German, Johanna means a gift from God. In the family and neighborhood everybody was talking that Johanna is very lucky, she will study in a college and become a big doctor. Actually, 1908 was very fortunate and important year for the freedom of women in Germany. Government for the first time in history, changed laws, and allowed women to study in college and Universities. Also the German parliament passed a legislation to allow women to become members of political parties and prestigious clubs. Though women were given new rights and freedom, liberalization was slow and old values still persisted.

The tough life of a sage of science

Unluckily, Elisabeth died in 1920; family members thought that her father, being a poor loco mechanic, might not look after Johanna. So she was sent to an orphanage. This was a great shock for the little Johanna, but it had one positive side also. Education up to higher level was totally free for orphans.

In 1926, Germany was slowly recovering from the after effects of the First World War. Economic conditions were improving. Scholars and scientists were developing new technologies in every field. One third of all Nobel Prizes were being given to German academics.

Deaconess at Kaiserswerth

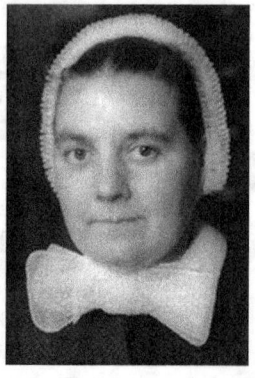

Johanna was very intelligent and sharp in studies from the beginning. In order to achieve good future, she decided to join the renowned Deaconess's Institute of Kaiserswerth in 1925. Theodor Fliedner, a pastor, founded Kaiserswerth Institute for welfare of unmarried mothers, prisoners, patients, orphans and poor children in 1836. In the beginning a Hospital and a Nursing School was established. This school was very famous Nursing School of that time. Florence Nightingale, known as mother of modern nursing, also studied in this Deaconess School in 1850. Intelligent Johanna easily got admission in this Institute. She was made a "deaconess" on March 30, 1932. This was the most appropriate place for her. There was a 1000 bedded hospital, pharmacy and a boarding school. She decided to study pharmacy.

After completing preliminary education in Kaiserswerth, she joined Münster University for further studies. Her analytical thinking and precise knowledge was noticed by her Professor Dr Hans Paul Kaufmann. He always encouraged and helped her. Here she passed state examination in pharmacy and was rewarded distinction in chemistry in 1936. Then she continued further education in physics, and received the title "Doctor of Science" at the University of Münster in 1938. On August 1, 1939, she was appointed as in-charge of pharmacy at the Military Hospital in Kaiserswerth.

Next month, Hitler's military forces attacked Poland. During war time, brave Johanna was busy in organizing and expanding the pharmacy. The war was not an easy time. There were two thousand people living in Kaiserswerth. Johanna was responsible for ensuring that there were enough medicines in this time of rationing and a thriving black market. She was well prepared and ready to fulfill any emergency demand for her patients. Many of her fellow deaconesses were often jealous and not co-operating but she continued evolving her professional skills. She was strong and was confronting every opponent (Dr. Johanna Budwig Stiftung).

Dr Budwig's scientific thinking, work and career

After Second World War, Johanna left Kaiserswerth in 1949. Soon Prof. Kaufmann came to know that she had left Kaiserswerth. He immediately met and persuaded her to work with him in Münster University, as he was always impressed from her talent. He converted the basement of his house into a laboratory and arranged all facilities for her research. He was famous as Fat Pope in the whole Europe.

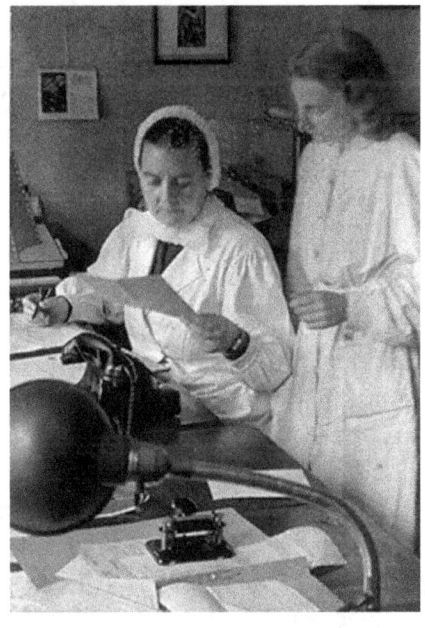

On Prof. Kaufmann's recommendation, Johanna was appointed as the chief expert for drugs and fats at the Federal Institute for Fats Research, Germany. This was the country's largest office issuing the approval of new drugs used for cancer. Many applications had been submitted to her for approval. These were the medications for cancer therapy with the sulfhydryl group (sulfur-containing protein compounds). Everywhere she saw that fats played a role in cellular respiration, also in expert reports provided by well-known professors like Prof. Nonnenbruch. Unfortunately, fats could only be detected in the late stage, and there were no method to distinguish between fats chemically.

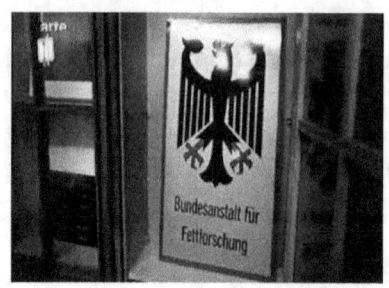

By this time, she developed paper chromatography. With this technique for first time she was able to detect fatty acids and lipoproteins directly even in 0.1 ml of blood. She used Co60 isotopes successfully to produce the first differential reaction for fatty acids, and produced the first direct iodine value via radioiodine. She also developed control of atmosphere in a closed system by using gas systems which act as antioxidants. She further developed Coloring methods, separating effects of fats and fatty acids. She too studied their behavior in blue and red light with fluorescent dyes.

Using rhodamine red dye, she studied the electrical behavior of the unsaturated fatty acids with their "halo". With this technique she could prove that electron rich highly unsaturated Linoleic and Linolenic fatty acids (Flax oil being the richest source) were the mysterious and undiscovered decisive fats required to attract oxygen into the cells, which Otto Warburg could not find. She studied the electromagnetic function of pi-electrons of the linolenic acid in the cell membranes, for nerve function, secretions, mitosis, as well as cell division. She also examined the synergism of the sulfur containing protein with the pi-electrons of the highly unsaturated fatty acids and their significance for the formation of the hydrogen bridge between fat and protein, which represent "the only path" for fast and focused Transport of electrons during respiration. This research was extensively

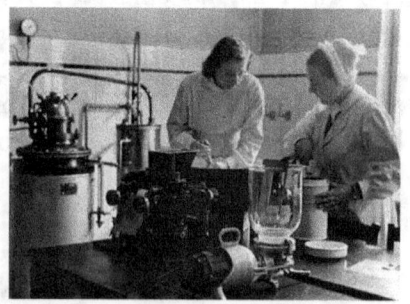

published in 1950 in Neue Wege in der Fettforschung (New Directions in Fat Research) and other publications.

This immediately caused an excitement and turmoil in the scientific community. Everybody thought that it would open new doors in Cancer research. She also proved that hydrogenated fats and refined oils including all Trans-fatty acids were not having vital electrons and were respiratory poisons.

During her research, she found that the blood of seriously ill cancer patients had deficiency of unsaturated essential fats (Linoleic and Linolenic fatty acids), lipoproteins, phosphatides, and hemoglobin. She also had noticed that cancer 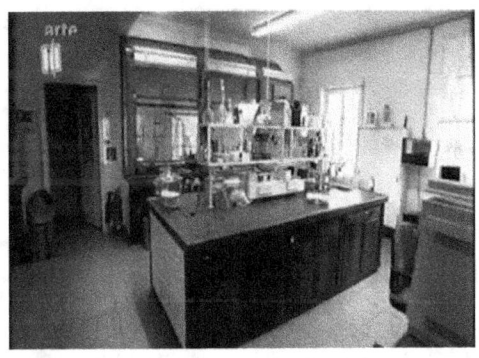 patients had a strange greenish-yellow substance in their blood which is not present in the blood of healthy people (Budwig, Cancer The Problem And The Solution).

She wanted to develop a healing program for cancer. So she enrolled over 642 cancer patients from four hospitals in Münster. She gave Flax oil and Cottage Cheeseto these patients. After just three months, patients began to improve in health and strength, the yellow green substance in their blood began to disappear, tumors gradually receded and at the same time the nutrients began to rise.

This way she developed a simple cure for cancer, based on the consumption of Flax oil with low fat Quark or cottage cheese, raw organic diet, mild exercise, Flax oil massage and the healing powers of the sun. It was a great victory and the first milestone in the battle against cancer. She treated approx. 2500 cancer patients during last few decades. Prof. Halme of surgery clinic in Helsinki used to keep records of her patients. According to him her success was over 90%, and this was achieved in cases, which were rejected by Allopathic doctors.

Dr. Budwig was a courageous scientist. She **loudly and convincingly argued that consumption of highly processed foods, particularly edible oils and margarines, which block the oxidation processes in the cells, are responsible for the development of cancer and other degenerative diseases.** She met with great resistance from food industry giants, who were doing everything to prevent the spread of her sensational discovery. In 1952, under the influence of strong pressure from this lobby, she lost her job and was barred from the research work.

Joins Medical School at Göttingen

Opponents of Dr. Johanna blamed her that she should not treat cancer patients because she doesn't have a doctor's degree. She felt this and eventually joined medical school in Göttingen in

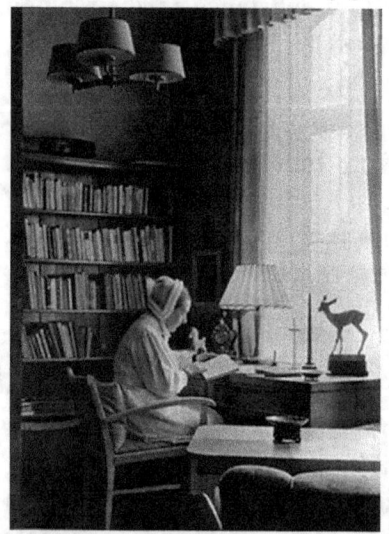

1955. Budwig was 47 years old at that time. She also continued her research work along with her studies. *Budwig successfully treated Prof. Martius's wife, who suffered from Breast Cancer*

One night a woman came with her small child whose arm was supposed to be amputated due to a tumor. She treated her and soon the amputation surgery was dismissed, and the child quickly did very well.

A Swiss woman came to her clinic in Göttingen. She suffered from Colon Cancer with metastasis and intestinal obstruction. Several doctors examined her, and was to be operated on Christmas Eve. On Budwig's request, she was treated by her protocol. The tumor of the colon quickly subsided. Seven weeks later, she was discharged without any detectable tumor. It is interesting that the Swiss custom officer was not ready to believe that the submitted passport belonged to same lady. Her look was so much changed! At home her daughter welcomed saying: "You look healthy, younger and more beautiful (from her book The Death of the Tumor – Vol. II).

After this, University allowed her to treat cancer patients with her oil-protein diet. She was getting miraculous results. University professors were excited with the results, but wanted that she should also include chemo and radiotherapy. She was rigid and didn't want to compromise. So she had differences and conflicts with her professors and ultimately left Göttingen (Budwig, Cancer The Problem And The Solution).

Last Destination - Dietersweiler-Freudenstadt

Eventually, she shifted to Dietersweiler-Freudenstadt, where she lived till her death. There she completed Ph.D. in Naturopathy so that she could legally treat cancer patients. She continued treating her patients in Freudenstadt. In 1968 she created unique Eldi oils for massage and enema, called Electron Differential Oils after performing precise spectroscopic measurements of the light absorption in different oils. *US pain institute has written somewhere: "What this crazy woman does with her ELDI oils, none of us manages to do via pain killers."*

Budwig conducted more than 200 lectures worldwide. Dr. Budwig was popular in the U.S. as FLAX SEED lady from Freudenstadt. She delivered her last public Lecture in Freudenstadt on March 3, 1999. On November 28, 2002, she fell down in her bathroom and got a fracture in right femur neck. She was admitted in a nursing home and ultimately died on May 19, 2003.

Budwig Protocol

The Budwig Protocol is one of the most widely followed alternative treatments for cancer and other diseases. The diet seems simple, but foods are powerful and can heal a person.

Transition Diet

The Transition diet is especially recommended for patients of liver, pancreatic or gall bladder cancers. The basic principle is that for 3 days nothing is eaten and drunk except the following written and at least three times daily warm tea (herbal teas from peppermint, rose hip, mallow or green tea) is drunk. Dr Budwig has recommended variant 1 for patients with a relatively good energy state, and variant 2 and 3 mainly for seriously ill patients.

Variant 1

Variant 1 for three days, 250 g of linomel or alternatively freshly crushed Flax seed is eaten together with the following:

- Freshly pressed fruit juices without added sugar.
- Freshly pressed vegetable juices such as carrot, celery juice, red beetroots and apple juice.
- Chinese tea and black tea are allowed in the morning
- Honey for sweetening is allowed. Just as grape juice for drinking and as a sweetner. Energetically weak patients can also consume sparkling wine and linomel.

Variant 2

For three days, oat meal cereal very hour with linomel is eaten daily with the following juices:

- Freshly pressed fruit juices or freshly pressed vegetable juices such as carrot, celery juice, beetroot and apple juice.
- Chinese tea and black tea are allowed in the morning.
- Honey for sweetening is allowed. Just as grape juice for drinking and as a sweetner.

- Energetically weak patients can also consume sparkling wine and linomel.

Variant 3

For three days, oatmeal soup with linomel is given three times a day together with the following juices:

- Freshly pressed fruit juices or fruit juices without added sugar.
- Freshly pressed vegetable juices such as carrot, celery juice, beetroot and apple juice.
- Chinese tea and black tea are allowed in the morning.
- Honey for sweetening is allowed. Just as grape juice for drinking and as a sweetner.
- Energetically weak patients can also consume sparkling wine and linomel.

It is often experienced frequently that patients mixed all three variants and "nevertheless" had good results. So better you to stick to one variant. (Budwig – Cancer The Problem And The Solution 2005: p.36).

Budwig Diet

The Budwig Protocol is necessary for many diseases from cancer to type 2 diabetes and heart disease to autoimmune diseases, etc. Its purpose is to energize the cells by restoring the natural electrical potential in the cell. Many human diseases are caused by "sick cells" which have lost their normal electrical potential; generally via a lower ATP energy in the cell's mitochondria.

6:00 AM – Sauerkraut juice

A glass of sauerkraut juice consumed before breakfast every morning. It is rich in vitamins including C, enzymes and helps develop the health-promoting gut flora. Sauerkraut is cabbage that has been pickled by natural fermentation, mainly with lactobacillus bacteria. It is slightly salty, sharp and sour. Well made, it is much nicer than it sounds. You may also consume another glass of sauerkraut juice later in the day.

It interesting that sauerkraut contains right rotating lactic acids and is highly alkaline and neutralizes levo-rotating lactic acids and makes our body alkaline. That is why Marcus Porcius Cato the Elder issued a statement - Carcinomas are incurable except with the treatment with Sauerkraut.

8:00 AM Breakfast

Green or herbal tea

Start breakfast with a cup of warm herbal or green tea. Sweeten with only natural honey. You can add lemon or grape juice. Patient should take such a tea before or with Linomel Muesli. You may consume 4-5 such teas in a day.

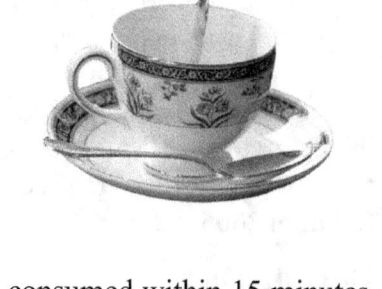

Linomel Muesli or Oil-Protein Muesli

This should be made fresh and consumed within 15 minutes. It is full of high energy pi-electrons, attract oxygen in the cells

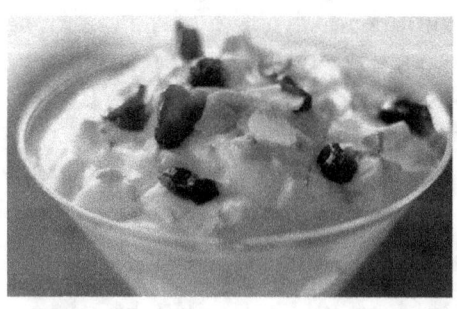

and capable of healing cell membranes. It is full of energy-rich omega-3 fats, has power to attract healing photons from sun through resonance. As "Om" is divine word and synonym of God in India. According to Hindu Mythology, the whole universe is located inside "Om", so the name Omkhand has been given to this wonderful recipe in Hindi.

Ingredients

- 3 Tbsp cold pressed organic Flax seed oil (FO)
- 100-125gm (6 Tbsp) Quark or Cottage Cheese(CC)

- 2 Tbsp freshly ground Flax seeds
- 2 Tbsp milk
- 1 cup fruits
- ¼ cup dried nuts
- Natural honey
- Flavorings – lemon, apple cider vinegar, cinnamon, pure cacao, natural vanilla, shredded coconut etc.

Recipe

Place 2 tablespoons Linomel or freshly ground Flax seeds in a small bowl. It is covered with raw, crushed or diced seasonal fruits depending on the season. Pour some orange or grape juice over this. Linomel™ is a brand name and originally created and patented by Budwig. It is a cereal made from cracked Flax Seed, a small amount of honey and a little milk powder.

Then the Quark-Flax seed oil cream is prepared in as follows: First add Flax seed oil, milk and honey and blend briefly with a hand-held immersion electric blender, then gradually add the Quark in smaller portions. Blend till oil and Quark is thoroughly mixed with no separated oil. Then it is seasoned differently everyday with different flavorings such as vanilla, cinnamon or various fruits such as banana, apple, lemon, orange juice, or berries.

Use various fruits such as fresh berries, apple, cherry, orange, banana, papaya, grapes etc. Add other fresh fruit if you like, totaling 1/2 to 1 cup of fruit. Budwig specially advised to use berries like strawberry, blueberry, raspberry, cheery

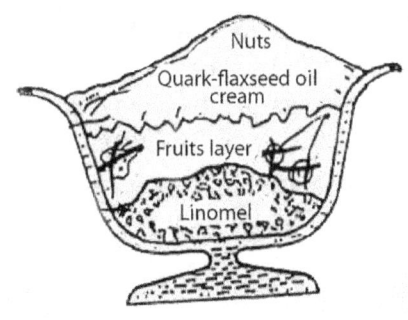

etc. because berries have ellagic acids which are strong cancer fighters.

Add organic raw nuts such as walnuts, almonds, raisins or Brazil nuts. They have sulfurated proteins, omega-3 fats and vitamins. Brazil nut is especially important because a single nut provides you with all of the selenium you need for the day. Selenium is very important to boost immune power. Peanuts are prohibited.

For variety and flavor, try natural vanilla, cinnamon, lemon juice, pure cocoa or shredded coconut.

Once blended in Budwig Cream, Quark and Flax seed oil form a new substance called lipoprotein. Lipoprotein is a water soluble complex. The Quark is rich in the sulfur-containing amino acids, methionine and cysteine. These positively charged amino acids attract the negatively charged electron clouds in fatty acid chains and exhibit a stabilizing effect on the highly unsaturated, otherwise easily oxidized fats. Thus, the amino acids protect the polyunsaturated fatty acids from the Flax seed oil against oxidation which, as a result, are able to enter the human body unchanged and with their full energy potential. The result: they are much more valuable to cells and their membranes. Consequently, one could say that Quark excels as a protector for the polyunsaturated fatty acids.

Sulfur-rich amino acids play a wealth of roles in many vital functions in our bodies. In combination with polyunsaturated fatty acids, they are important partners in regulating the uptake of oxygen and its utilization by the cell. They therefore contribute significantly to a strong immune system, healthy metabolism, and mental vitality. For many generations, people have been getting their omega-3 fatty acids from fish, vegetables, nuts, and seeds. Our health literally depends on the regular consumption of the essential omega-3 and omega-6 fatty acids, alpha-linolenic acid (ALA) and linoleic acid (LA). Our bodies require these fatty acids in order to synthesize their cell membranes as well as for a variety of metabolic processes and heal the cancer and other diseases.

Tips for making the Budwig Mixture

- Follow directions properly! It is important to add things to the mixture in the right order. If you mix them in the wrong order you may lose a lot of the opportunity to convert the oil-soluble omega-3 into water soluble-omega-3.

- Keep the Flax seed oil refrigerated.
- Immersion blender is a must.
- The mixture can be flavored differently every day by adding nuts and fruits preferably organic such as pecans, almonds or walnuts (not peanuts), banana, organic cocoa, shredded coconut, pineapple (fresh) blueberries, raspberries, cinnamon, vanilla or (freshly) squeezed fruit juice.
- Consume immediately for best results.

10 AM Vegetable juice

Freshly squeezed vegetable juice from carrots, beets, celery, tomato, and radish, lemon as well as green vegetables - stinging nettle, lettuce or spinach. Apple is added to sweeten and enhance the taste. Carrot & beet juices are especially helpful to the liver and have strong cancer fighting properties. Vary vegetables. Some tasty and nutritious combinations are beet and apple juice, carrot and apple, carrot and beet, asparagus and apple, celery and apple, celery and carrot. Beet juice should not be taken alone. If taken alone it may cause red or pink urine (beeturia).

She also frequently recommended the following juices:

1. Nettle juice - Especially in the spring, Dr Budwig recommended to puree nettles with water and a lemon.

2. Radish juice - For this, a radish is first crushed and then thrown together with a lemon into the juicer. This juice is by the way durable for several days and Dr Budwig has sometimes recommended her patients to drink a small quantity of them every day.

3. Coltsfoot juice - For this juice, with the exception of the harder old rootstock, the entire remaining underground shoot is mixed with a few flowers and some milk and honey.

4. Horseradish juice - Mix 3-5 cm horseradish together with an apple and (raw) milk. Depending on the quantity of milk you can change the taste. Dr Budwig recommended this juice above all to workmen and to stimulate the appetite. Freshly pressed means, by the way, that you drink the juice within 5 minutes after pressing. In some cases, Dr Budwig prescribed a second juice 30 to 60 minutes later.

12:15 PM Lunch

Salad Platter: Salad plate with homemade cottage cheese-Flax seed mayonnaise. As salad also use: dandelion, cress, celery, tomato, cucumber, lettuce, radish, cabbage, broccoli, green horseradish and pepper.

Delicious mayo salad dressing can be prepared by mixing together 2 Tbsp (30 ml) Flax Oil, 2 Tbsp (30 ml) milk, and 2 Tbsp (30 ml) cottage cheese. Then add 2 tablespoons (30 ml) of Lemon juice (or Apple Cider Vinegar) and add 1 teaspoon (2.5 g) Mustard powder plus some herbs of your choice. Other alternative dressing can be made by mixing Flax Oil, lemon juice, Mustard and some herbs (Budwig, The Oil-Protein Diet Cookbook, 1994).

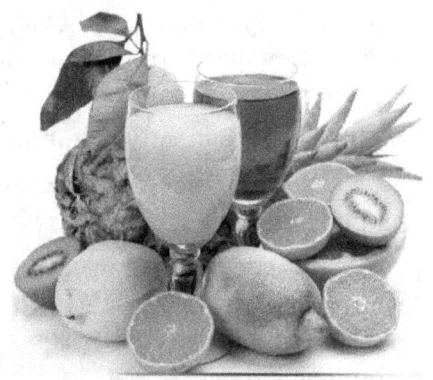

Main Course: Vegetables cooked in water, then flavored with Oleolox and herbs possibly with oatmeal, soy sauce, curry etc. Vegetable broth flavored with a little Oleolox and yeast flakes. As side dish for the vegetables: buckwheat, brown rice, millet or potatoes can be used. One or two slices of Ezekiel bread can be taken. Use lot of dried fruits in the main meal also.

Lunch Dessert: Cottage cheese/ Flax oil mixture served as a dessert, prepared with dry fruits and fruits such as apple, or poured over a fruit salad. You already know how to prepare it

74

perfectly. You will find wonderful recipes for a delicious dessert in the Oil-Protein cookbook by Budwig. Please note that the dessert is **"a must"** and should definitely be eaten. So keep your main course light so you may enjoy the dessert happily.

The form of preparation as "fruit foam," "Linovita" or "red coat in the snow" (in Oil-Protein cookbook) is always welcoming for the healthy and the sick. In all the gimmicks in the preparation of the delicious desserts, one should be aware: Quark and Flaxseed give the patient immense power within a short space of time. Always fresh and beautiful, always freshly interesting, this important food for life should be for the sick and for the whole family.

3 PM Fruit juices

In the afternoon, Dr Budwig recommended different kinds of fruit juices e.g. apples, grapes, cherries, pineapples, papaya, or apricot, sparkling wine or wine - with or without Flaxseeds or with or without a few drops Flaxseed oil.

Budwig preferred papaya juice and recommended her patients to drink at least every 2 days a glass of papaya juice. The main reason for this was definitely the protein splitting enzyme papain.

6 PM Dinner

The evening meal should be light and served early, around 6 p.m. A warm meal may be prepared using brown rice, buckwheat or oat meal. Never consume corn or soy beans. Dishes made with buckwheat grouts are most easily tolerated and nourishing. Use only honey to sweeten. Soup or more solid dishes can be combined with a tasty sauce according to preference. Use OLEOLOX liberally also to sweet sauces and soups, making them nourishing and a richer source of energy.

8:30 PM

A glass of organic red wine may be consumed. All things are a matter of correct dosage. This glass of red wine is not a "must" program. In fact, seriously ill patients having pain and discomfort just starting on the oil-protein diet, it is recommended to serve a glass of red wine mixed with freshly ground Flax seeds to tide them over while going off pain killers (Budwig, Cancer The Problem And The Solution).

METRIC CONVERSION TABLE	
10 g = 0.35 oz	5 cc = 1 teaspoon
100 g = 3.5 oz	15 cc = 1 tablespoon
150 g = 5.25 oz	30 cc = 1 ounce
250 g = 8.8 oz	250 cc = 1 cup
454 g = 1 lb	960 cc = 1 qt
Oz = ounce lb = pound qt = quart Tsp = teaspoon Tbsp = tablespoon	

Precautions

Drink filtered water - Use RO (Reverse Osmosis)water for drinking, cooking and enemas.

Eat Organic Diet - Always try to eat organic food.

Dental Care –

Mercury is a Carcinogenic as well as a Poison! The root canals of dead teeth are full of bacteria that attack the liver and lymphatic system. From Amalgam fillings the mercury slowly leaks out of the filings. The ADA cleverly defends the use of amalgam in spite of the fact that there is sufficient evidence that patients with many severe problems, including psychotic episodes and fatal allergic reactions, were just cured by removing the amalgam. It is advisable to rather have a ceramic filling than be slowly poisoned by mercury. Even gold filling is dangerous; it acts as battery producing electrical current. Be informed that the effect of drugs, including poison, is dose dependant and cumulative.

Fluoride is not only toxic but it is also carcinogenic. Fluoride has never been proven to prevent tooth decay. It has been outlawed in many countries or groups of countries because the evidence is overwhelming that fluoride causes premature aging, so drink bottled water and use fluoride-free toothpaste (American Cancer Institute - 1963).

I highly recommend helping you avoid fillings in the first place. Holistic dentist recommend 3% H_2O_2 as a gargle or rinse, or making a paste using baking soda. H_2O_2 usage three times a day is advised. It is great for cleaning dentures, too.

Frying and deep frying - Frying and deep frying is not allowed
to cook patient's food. Never heat any oil in the kitchen. By heating oils the wealth of high energy electrons is destroyed and Trans fats and dangerous toxic chemicals such as acrylamides are

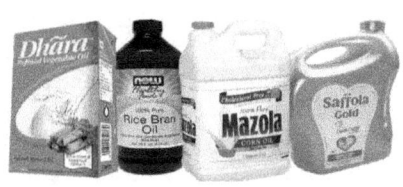

formed in the oil. Boiling and steaming are good practices. You can fry vegetables etc. in water and add oleolox before serving. Water is the safest medium for frying, says Lothar Hirneise.

Chemo and Radio -

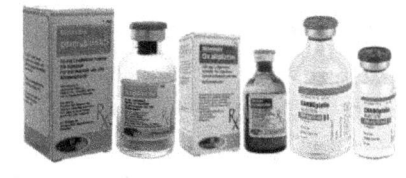

Chemotherapy is aimed at destruction of the tumor, and it destroys many living cells, and the entire person. Anything that disturbs growth is fatal because growth is an elementary function of life. We cannot achieve something good with bad tools.

Dr. Budwig rejects Chemo and Radiation Therapy. Budwig used to say with full confidence and clarity, "My treatment targets on the real cause of cancer; it fills cancer cells with high energy pi-electrons and attracts oxygen into the cells. And cancer cells start to breathe and produce vital energy."

Man-made Supplements - With this treatment man-made antioxidants, synthetic vitamins and pain killers should not be given. The dose of anticoagulants and aspirin should be adjusted by your doctor. Dr. Budwig favors natural, herbal and homeopathy instead of man-made and synthetic supplements, vitamins and pain killers (Budwig, Cancer The Problem And The Solution).

Prohibitions of Budwig Protocol

In this protocol there are certain restrictions. They are as important as the diet itself. It is very difficult to defeat the cancer without strictly following these rules.

Sugar is strictly forbidden

Sugar, Jiggery, molasses, maple syrup and artificial sweeteners like xylitol, aspartame are not permitted. You can use only natural honey, stevia and fruit juices – all off course unprocessed.

Avoid meats, eggs and fish

Meat, fish, poultry, eggs, and butter are never allowed. Preserved meat is like a poison. It is highly processed and treated with dangerous antibiotics, preservatives and nitrates.

Stop using Hydrogenated Fat and Refined oil

You can never eat pizza, burger, fast food, fried food, biscuits etc. as they all are made by hydrogenated margarine and shortenings. Hydrogenation is a very dangerous process, used to increase shelf life of fats. In this process (oil is heated at very high temperature and hydrogen is passed through oils in presence of nickel) killing Trans fats are formed, high energy live and vital electrons are destroyed and nutrients are damaged. Hydrogenated Fats is just a dead, nutrition-less and cancer causing liquid plastic. Budwig always preached against these damaging fats. She has allowed low fat cheese, oleolox and coconut oil.

Preservatives and Processed Food

You should not eat Potato chips, soft drinks etc. which are full of preservatives. Never consume highly processed food e.g. ready to eat packed foods, pasta, pastries, bread and soy products, tofu etc. However good quality soy souse is permitted.

Microwave, Teflon, Aluminum and Plastic

Never cook in microwave oven. Food cooked in microwave become toxic and deformed. Also don't use aluminum, plastic, Teflon coated cookware and aluminum foils. Use stainless steel, iron, china clay or glass utensils instead.

Chemicals and pesticides are not allowed

Avoid pesticides and chemicals, even those in household products & cosmetics. Stay away from mosquito repellants, sun screen lotions and sun glasses.

Wear natural fibers

Don't wear clothes made using synthetic fiber like nylon, polyester and acrylic. Budwig put great emphasis on the fact that her patients only wore natural fabrics such as cotton or satin, since they too can influence the magnetic field of our body.

Bed

Don't use on foam pillow and mattress. She recommended horsehair mattresses. Latex mattresses are the second choice. In any case, however, you should always replace mattresses that have metal spring cores.

CRT TV and mobile phones

These emit dangerous electromagnetic radiation, so do not use them. You can watch LCD and plasma TVs.

No left over

Food should be prepared fresh and eaten soon after preparation to maximize intake of health giving electrons and enzymes (Budwig, Cancer The Problem And The Solution).

Few Desserts recipes by Dr. Budwig

Fujiya delight

Ingredients for 3 people:
> 250 cc grape juice, 250 cc pure currant juice,
> 8g agar-agar, Quark-Flaxseed oil,
> Milk, honey, vanilla cream

Preparation:

Heat the grape juice till it boils, then add the currant juice, agar-agar, stirring constantly for 5 minutes, and allow to cool. Now divide this mass to 3 narrow, tall cups, which have been rinsed with cold water. It is preferable if these cups have a bottom diameter of only 3- 4 cm. Refrigerate to cool. Now mix a Quark-Flaxseed oil cream with milk, honey and vanilla. Turn the red jelly upside down onto glass plates. The Quark-Flaxseed oil cream is placed on the top so that only the upper half is covered with the Quark-Flaxseed oil cream, so that top looks like the Snow caped Mount Fujiyama.

(The beautiful hotel with a gorgeous view of the Fujiyama is called "Fujiya", hence the dessert "Fujiya".)

Linovita-in-love in wine jelly

Ingredients: for 5 people:
> 250 cc of grape juice, 250 ccm of white wine,
> 8 agar-agar, 4 tablespoons of milk,
> 8 tablespoons of Flaxseed oil, 2 teaspoons of honey,
> 200-250 g of Quark, 2 liqueur glasses
> Vodka, plum (Slibowitz) or cherry brandy or rum

Preparation:

The wine jelly is prepared by heating 250 cc of grape juice till it boils. Agar-agar is stirred with a little wine and placed in the boiling grape juice. Immediately remove from the cooking plate and add the remaining wine gradually with constant stirring.

After about 5 minutes, the jelly mixture clears itself. You can now divide to approx. 5 glass bowls or champagne glasses. Immediately afterwards, mix the Quark-Flaxseed oil cream from Flaxseed oil, milk, honey and Quark. Finally, add 2 liqueur glasses of vodka or slibovitz or cherry brandy or rum into the Quark-Flaxseed oil cream. This Quark-Flaxseed oil mixture is evenly divided on the ready to-use bowls so that the Quark-Flaxseed oil cream partly sinks down in the middle. It is served after complete solidification.

(Oil-Protein Diet by Lothar Hirneise available at http://www.hirneise.com/page-8/page-19/)

Ice cream with cocoa

Ingredients:
   3 tablespoons of Flaxseed oil, 3 tablespoons of milk,
   1 tablespoon of honey, 100g of Quark, 100 g of hazelnuts,
   2 tablespoons of cocoa

Preparation:
   Quark, Flaxseed oil, milk and honey are mixed in the blender, then the hazelnuts are added, well blended and finally, cocoa is added to the mixture. Now pour the entire mixture into the ice-maker and place it in the fridge compartment of the refrigerator. This mixture with a nougat flavor gives the various combinations mentioned here the dark color contrast. For very ill people these preparations are very important, especially when there is a general lack of appetite.

(Oil-Protein Diet by Lothar Hirneise available at http://www.hirneise.com/page-8/page-19/)

ELDI oils

Dr. Budwig created unique ELDI oils, called electron differential oils after performing precise spectroscopic measurements of the light absorption in different oils - specifying that the oils contained pi-electron clouds from Flax oil, wheat germ oil plus vitamin-E in its natural complex, etheric oils and sulfhydryl groups.

Dr. Johanna Budwig said, "The sun is my preferred treatment modality, as is ELDI oil, used externally to stimulate the absorption of the long-wave band of the sun. I have used ELDI oils extensively since 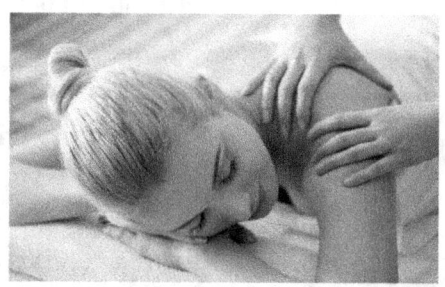 1968 for body massage as well as in the selective application of oil packs. US pain institute has written somewhere: "What this crazy woman does with her ELDI oils, none of us manages to do via pain killers." Dr. Budwig has mentioned that if ELDI oil is not available, you may use Flax oil instead. *You can buy ELDI oils at: www.sensei.de*

Massage Benefits

- Since ancient time massage has been part of cancer healing. Think of your lymphatics as a trash-disposal system for your body. Massage initiates lymphatic drainage, you push the trash out of your body and you're helping your immune system.
- Massage therapy is sometimes the first really pleasant touch a patient is able to experience.
- Massage also releases endorphins (our body's natural painkillers), stimulates lymph movement, and stretches tissues throughout the body. It's energizing, stimulating, and pretty good feeling.

ELDI oil plans:

A: For cancer patients in support of the energy level

1. Full-body rubbings in the morning
2. ELDI oil R enema with 200ml every 2-3 days
3. Wrap at the "place of the happening"

B: For energetically weak patients

1. Full-body rubbings in the morning and in the evening
2. Enema: standard plan for ELDI oil R
3. Wrap at the "place of the happening"
4. Daily liver wrap with ELDI oil sage

Additional information:

- Make sure that you make once a week an (deep/high) enema with water or coffee.
- If you make daily coffee enemas, then start in the morning with the coffee enema and then with the ELDI R enema, but only if your energetic level allows you to make two enemas daily. Otherwise, only make the ELDI R enema. (Oil Protein Diet by Lothar Hirneise)

ELDI oils from SENSEI (www.sensei.de) are produced in a permanent cold chain in a European oil mill and marketed under the name of Electron Differentiation Oils. There are two qualities. A 6-star organic quality and a 5-star quality, which are produced exclusively for the IOPDF (www.iopdf.com).

Cost factor ELDI oils

Again and again we hear that for reasons of cost, patients use Flax seed oil instead of ELDI oil R for an enema. Please do not do so, because Flax seed oil does not react in the same way as ELDI oil R. Instead, use cheap ELDI oils from IOPDF or reduce the amount of oil.

Procedure –

Two times a day, i.e. morning and evening, rub ELDI Oil or Flax oil into the skin over the whole body, a bit more intensely on the shoulders, armpits and groin area (where plenty of lymphatic vessels are present) as well as the problem areas, such as the breast, stomach, liver, etc. Leave the oil on the skin for about 20 minutes and follow with a warm water shower without washing with soap. After 10 minutes take another shower, this time using a mild soap, and then relax for 15-20 minutes.

Once the body has been oiled and the ELDI Oil or Flax oil has penetrated the skin, the warm water will open the skin pores and the oil penetrates the skin more deeply. The second shower, where one washes with soap, cleanses the skin so that clothes and linen will not become overly soiled.

Oil Packs

Take a piece of cloth made of pure cotton. Cut to a size to fit the body part, such as the knee. Soak the cotton cloth with oil, place on the knee etc., cover it with a piece of polythene and wrap it up with an elastic bandage. Leave overnight. Remove in the morning and wash the knee; repeat in the evening. Keep applying the same procedure for weeks, you get good results. You also use Flax oil or castor oil for these local applications if you do not get ELDI oils . Dr Budwig generally recommended ELDI sage and should be used in the following indications:

- Tumors
- Painful skin areas
- Metastases
- Hepatic impairment and liver support
- Kidney problems
- Bladder disorders
- Intestinal cramps
- Lung disorders
- Bone disorders of all kinds

ELDI Oil Enema

Enemas are used in the Oil-Protein Diet exclusively for the energy intake and not for the purification of the intestine. Dr Budwig used to give ELDI oil or Flax oil enema to her serious

84

patients. Budwig used to get immediate and miraculous results with the most seriously ill patients. Flax seed Oil enema also give similar results.

I recommend you to make the first enemas only with 100ml and then increase over several days to 250ml. Some patients have enemas with 500ml oil and positively reported on it. 500ml are however the absolute exception and mostly not necessary. Usually 250ml suffice.

Incidentally, smaller amounts are also easily introduced with an enema syringe instead of with an enema bucket. Enema syringes are available in sizes up to 350ml and are easy to handle.

Standard plan for ELDI oil R: Day 1 = 100ml, day 2 = 100ml, day 3 = 150ml, day 4 = 150ml, day 5 = 200ml, day 6 = 200ml and day 7 = 250ml.

From the seventh day, one remains at 250ml, and so long until the patient is significantly better. Then you can go back to 100ml - 150ml, always together with 1-2 daily whole body rubbings. (Oil Protein Diet by Lothar Hirneise)

Ingredients

- Enema pot
- Watch
- A bowl to collect oil when you are getting rid of bubbles.
- Towel and tissue
- RO filtered water
- ELDI oil or Flax oil
- Towel or Drip Stand

Procedure

Prepare a place near the toilet, so that if you can't hold the enema, you will be making a quick dash and the shorter distance is better.

Cleansing Enema with Plain water

First of all you should take a plain water enema. Purpose of this enema is cleaning of intestines. It is not a retention enema and is evacuated immediately. For this you may use 500-1000ml (2-4 cups) RO filtered water. As soon as the whole water is inside the rectum, go and sit on the commode and release the water slowly.

Take the oil enema immediately after the water enema

- Use advised (above) amount of ELDI or Flax oil. The oil should be at body temperature. The best test is to dip your little finger into the oil.
- Fill the oil into the enema pot. It takes at least 5 minutes for the bubbles to get out of the tube.
- The enema pot should be hanged on a drip stand about 2-3 feet above your body.
- You need to lubricate the nozzle and anus with Flax oil. When all is ready, lie on your right side in the fetal position. Insert the nozzle into the rectum slowly and carefully with your left hand, and un-pinch the tube.
- If you feel little uncomfortable when the oil is going in, pinch the tube, wait till the feeling passes away, then continue again.
- The oil is much more viscous and moves more slowly. You might need to hold the pot a bit higher to get it to run a bit quicker.
- Once the oil is in, wait and hold it for about 12 minutes. After that slowly turn yourself to left side and hold oil for another 12 minutes. You may listen to music while taking enema.
- When done, it is best to sit on the commode for about 15 minutes with something to read (Skelton).

Coffee Enema

Dr. Max Gerson introduced coffee enema back in the 1930s. In this enema about 500ml of coffee is pushed into rectum, this amount only reaches up to sigmoid colon. There is no loss of minerals and electrolytes in Coffee Enema because their absorption occurs well before sigmoid colon. Coffee enema is even safe for those who are allergic to coffee because it is not absorbed into the systemic circulation. You may take this enema once or twice. It has the following benefits:

- **Powerful and Natural Pain Reliever**
- **Cleansing** - Coffee also acts as an astringent in the large intestine, helps cleanse the colon walls.
- **Toxin Elimination** - The major benefit of the coffee enema is elimination of toxins through the liver. Caffeine, theophylline and theobromine dilate the blood vessels and bile ducts, stimulate the liver to discharge more bile and boost the detoxifying process into high gear and heal inflammation. Indeed, endoscopic studies confirm they increase bile output.
- **Stimulates Liver** - Kahweol and cafestol palmitate found in coffee promote the activity of a key enzyme system called glutathione S-Transferase. This is an important mechanism in the detoxification of carcinogens, as the enzyme group is responsible for neutralizing free radicals. Coffee enema stimulates the activity of this system by 600- 700%.

Coffee Enema Procedure
- This enema is retained for 12-14 minutes, during this time blood circulates in liver three times and blood is purified. Coffee enema can be given several times a day, few patients take up to seven times a day. Normally if pain is not relieved it may be taken more than one time. You should relax while taking enema; you may listen to music or read newspaper while relaxing. The best time for coffee enema is either early morning after you passed motion or during the day time.

- Grind organic coffee beans. Put approx. 750ml of filtered water in a steal pan and bring it to boil. Add 2-5 heaped Tbsp coffee powder, 3 Tbsp is ideal. It is roughly 20-25grams. Let it continue to simmer for ten minutes or more and then turn off the burner. Allow it to cool down to a very comfortable, tepid temperature. Test it with your finger. It should be the same temperature as your body's temperature. Filter the coffee with fine mesh steal sieve into a jug. This is approximately 500ml.
- Pour 2 cups (500ml) of coffee into the enema pot. Be sure the plastic hose is clamped tightly. Now open the clamp and grasp, but do not close the clamp on the hose. Place the enema tip in the sink. Hold up the enema bag above the tip until the coffee begins to flow out. As soon as it starts flowing, quickly close the clamp. This expels any air in the tube.
- Lubricate the enema tip with a small amount of coconut oil or KY jelly. Create a comfortable and relaxing atmosphere. After a few days you will thoroughly enjoy this ritual.
- Light a candle, play some light music and most importantly, make sure you are comfortable and warm. We recommend placing a pillow with a washable cover under your head and lying down on a old towel.
- The position preferred is lying on your back. With the clamp closed hang the pot about 3 feet above your belly. We like to hang the enema pot on a drip stand.
- Insert the tip gently into anus and open the clamp slowly. You should relax and breathe. The coffee may take a few seconds to begin flowing. If you develop a cramp, close the hose clamp, turn from side to side and take a few deep breaths. The cramp will usually pass quickly. Usually nothing happens.
- When all the liquid is inside, close the clamp and remove it slowly. Retain the enema for 12- 14 minutes. You may remain lying on the floor.

- After 14 minutes or so, go to the toilet and empty your gut. Take your time. Wash the enema pot and tube thoroughly with soap and water.
- Take more potassium in the form of fruits and vegetable juices if you take coffee enema regularly (S.A.Wilsons.com).

Epsom bath

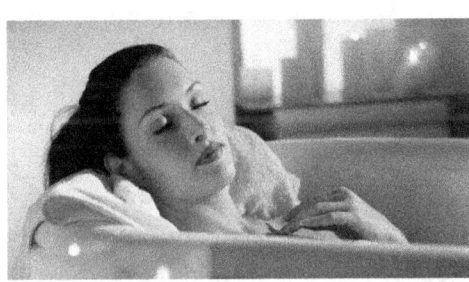

Detoxification of your body through bathing is an ancient remedy that anyone can perform in the comfort of your own home. Your skin is known as the third kidney, and toxins are excreted through sweating. An Epsom salt bath is thought to assist your body in eliminating toxins as well as absorbing the magnesium and nutrients that are in the water. Soaking in Epsom salt actually helps replenish the body's magnesium levels, combating hypertension. The sulfate flushes toxins and helps form proteins in brain tissue and joints. Most of all, it will leave you relaxed, refreshed and awakened. Take it once a week or as advised.

Prepare your bath

- It is a 40 minutes ritual. The first 20 minutes are said to help your body remove the toxins, while the second 20 minutes are for absorbing the minerals from the water
- Fill your tub with comfortably hot water. Use a chlorine filter if possible.
- Add Epsom salt (Magnesium sulfate). For people 50 Kg and up, add 2 cups or more to a standard bath tub.
- Then add 2 cups or more of soda bicarb. It is known for its cleansing ability and even has anti-fungal properties. It also leaves skin very soft.

- Add 2-3 Tbsp ground ginger. While this step is optional, ginger can increase your heat levels, helping to sweat out more toxins. However, since it is heating the body, it may cause your skin to turn slightly red for a few minutes, so be careful with the amount you add. Depending on the capacity of your tub, anywhere from 1 Tbsp to 1/3 cup can be added (Herneise).
- Add aromatherapy oils. Again optional, but there are many oils that will make the bath an even more pleasant and relaxing experience (such as lavender), as well as those that will assist in the detoxification process (tea tree or eucalyptus oil). Around 20 drops is sufficient for a standard bath.
- Swish all of the ingredients around in the tub, and then slip into the tub. You should start sweating within the first few minutes. If you feel too hot, start adding cold water into the tub until you cool off.
- Get out of the tub slowly and carefully. Your body has been working hard and you may get lightheaded or feel weak and drained. On top of that, the salts make your tub slippery, so stand with care.
- Drink plenty of water and relax in bed for a few minutes

Soda bicarb bath

Lothar Hirneise has given lot of importance to Soda bicarb bath. It is thought to assist you in eliminating toxins as well as making your body alkaline so your tumor cells may suffocate. Patient may take it once or even twice a day. Just add 2 cups of soda bicarb in your bath tub filled with warm water and relax in it for 30-40 minutes (Hirneise, 2005).

Sun Therapy

Getting an adequate amount of sunshine is a critical part of Budwig protocol. Once the body has acquired the right oil-protein balance with the Cottage Cheeseand Flax oil, the body develops better capacity to absorb the healing photons from the sun. Remember that for healing of cancer high energy photons from the sun are very important. The sunshine is important to maintain adequate vitamin-D levels in our body. Vitamin-D is a powerful antioxidant that has been linked to preventing many diseases including cancer.

Dr. Budwig's focus was on the importance of photons from the sunbeams and their interaction with vital essential fats (linoleic and linolenic acid) in our body. It is the interaction of photons from the sun and the electrons in proper food that provide the synergistic effect on healing our body. Eating the electron rich Flax oil/Cottage Cheesemixture, must be connected with adequate exposure to sunlight.

There is nothing else on earth with a higher concentration of photons of the sun's energy than man. This concentration of the sun's energy is very much energetic point for humans, with their wave eminently suitable lengths - is improved when we eat electron rich essential oils, which in turn absorbs the photons in the form of electro-magnetic waves of sunbeams.

When you eat the FO/CC mixture, your body becomes a better antenna for the photons from the sunbeam. Your body develops a better ability to absorb the energy from the sun and Transfer it to your cells to perform their vital functions. You become energized at a deep level, and when this happens cancer is healed itself.

It is red light that penetrates deeper in the tissues. In 1968 Dr. Budwig used 695 nm ruby (red) laser light with success to radiate healthy surrounding cancer tissues in cancer patients.

Oil-Protein Diet while travelling

- In her Oil-Protein Diet Cookbook, Dr. Budwig writes: "While traveling, you can always care for yourself with Linomel and hot or cold milk, and/or fruit juices."

- If you are eating a salad in a restaurant, never take the finished dressings, but use olive oil and vinegar. The chance not to take Trans fats is at the least.
- If you want something to be fried, ask the cook to put it in coconut fat or butter. Butter is present in every kitchen.
- Budwig also recommends eating various types of fresh fish to replace the Flax oil and Quark when travelling. You can protect yourself against harm while travelling by ordering fresh fish such as trout, pike, carp and other fresh fish. However, canned (tinned) fish, also shrimps, prawn and other items which frequently contain artificial coloring agents and harmful chemical preservatives, must be strictly avoided.
- Do not eat the "muesli" in hotels. They are mostly denatured carbohydrates.
- Do not use polyunsaturated oils (Flax seed oil, Oil, pumpkin seed oil, etc.) which are kept at room temperature and all contain Trans fatty acids.

For a long vacation

During your long stay travelling away from home, it is really simple to keep up with the Budwig diet, all that is needed was a little bit of preplanning. You may have a fridge and electric tea kettle in the hotel room, or you carry a ice chest.

Wash all fruits and veggies and make enough juice for the travel day and one more day. You should carry a bowl, fork, spoon, sharp knife, and hand blender, nuts, oatmeal and tea. You carry Flax oil, cottage cheese, fruits and veggies in a ice chests for travel.

If you have "eaten something", especially too many carbohydrates in the form of potatoes, rice, noodles or even a "not so healthy dessert/cake", then you should take a walk immediately after eating. (Healing Cancer Naturally)

Making Quark

Quark is a very popular and delicious cheese in Germany. You may find many recipes of making Quark on Google. I am giving you a simple recipe here. In this recipe you will learn how it is easy to make your own homemade Quark.

Ingredients

- 1 liter milk preferably <2% fat
- 500ml cultured buttermilk
- Cheese cloth

Instructions

- In a large glass bowl add milk and buttermilk. Stir well and cover with a clean kitchen towel.
- Let this sit at room temperature for 24 hours. The mixture will thicken slightly.
- Heat the oven to 125^0 F and shut off. Set the bowl uncovered into the oven for about 45 min. The mixture will change to yogurt like texture.
- Add a Cheese cloth to a colander and set on a large bowl.
- Pour the milk mixture into the colander, twist the ends and let drain for about 1 ½ to 2 hours.
- The Quark will be in the towel and the whey will be in the bowl. One liter milk usually yields 200gms of Quark.

Making Cottage Cheese

In some places good quality Cottage Cheeseis also not available and you need to make your own. Today I am giving you a very good recipe for home made cottage cheese.

Ingredients

- 1 liter natural, low-fat cow's milk preferably <2% fat
- 1/3 cup Vinegar
- Cold water

Instructions

- Mix 1/3 cup of vinegar in 2 cups of water and keep aside. Diluted vinegar yields soft cheese. You may also use diluted lemon juice.
- Boil the milk in a heavy bottomed pan over medium heat, stirring frequently making sure milk does not burn on the bottom of the pan. As the milk comes to a boil, remove the pan from the gas burner and place it on kitchen counter.
- Now add about a glass of cold water to bring the milk's temperature down to about 75-80 degrees Celsius. We want to curdle the milk at this temperature, so we get a soft cheese.
- Then add little (about 1-2 Tbsp) diluted vinegar slowly and stir the milk gently. After 10 seconds, add little vinegar slowly and stir the milk. Go on adding vinegar until the curd will start separating from the whey. Remember you should curdle the milk slowly.
- Once the cheese has completely separated from the whey, add a glass of cold water and drain the whey using a stainless steel strainer.
- Now Transfer the curdled cheese into a suitable container and blend thoroughly with electric hand blender until you get very smooth and thick creamy cheese. If the cheese is dry, add a little milk while blending. This is your home made cottage cheese.

Buckwheat

Dr. Budwig highly recommended buckwheat in her healing diet. Contrary to its name, this seed is not related to wheat. Buckwheat is a gluten free power food!

Buckwheat is supercharged with health-boosting nutrients and phytochemicals, including B-vitamins, magnesium, manganese, phosphorus, zinc, copper, potassium, and selenium. It is also one of the best natural sources of rutin and D-chiro-

Inositol, two phytochemicals that have been associated with a number of interesting health benefits. It is the best source of high-quality, easily digestible proteins. This makes it an excellent meat substitute. What's more, buckwheat grouts (the hulled kernels) are generally well tolerated and rarely cause allergic reactions or other adverse effects in humans. These gluten-free kernels can be served as an alternative to rice or made into delicious buckwheat porridge.

Studies have shown that populations eating diets high in fiber-rich whole grains and seeds, like buckwheat, consistently have lower risk for colon cancer. Research reported at the American Institute for Cancer Research (AICR) International Conference on Food, Nutrition and Cancer, by Rui Hai Liu, M.D., Ph.D., and his colleagues at Cornell University shows that buckwheat, contain many powerful phytonutrients that can fight cancer.

Energy Healing

Mild exercise

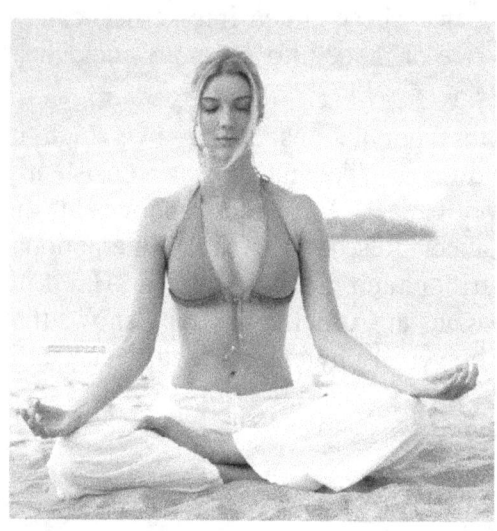

Patient can do mild exercise and remain active if his condition permits. He can go for a walk or do light yoga in the open terrace or garden under the healing and refreshing sunshine. Patient can jog for a few minutes after lunch or dinner. It is very beneficial for cancer patient. But if patient is serious and has metastasis, he should not jog, better he should relax in his house.

Patient can keep himself busy in many activities like sitting in garden enjoying nature, visualization, listening music, reading, laughing, chatting with friends etc. Stress, depression, anxiety, anger and fear can be very damaging to him. Share your feelings with your life partner or a best friend.

You should try your best to remove stress and negative thoughts and balance the flow of energy "prana" or "chi" in your body. Do meditation, Emotional Freedom Technique EFT, Qigong, Reiki, Acupuncture, Acupressure, Sun Salutation etc. to heal your body, mind and spirit.

Meditation

Meditation is a means of Transforming the mind. Meditation practices are techniques that encourage and develop concentration, clarity, positivity, and relaxation of the body and mind. Do any simple meditation for relaxation. Meditation stimulates pineal gland (*piyush granthi*) to shower melatonin hormone. Melatonin controls circadian rhythm and induces restorative sleep. Its powerful antioxidant effect offers important enhancements to the brain and nervous system, helping protect against age-related damage. Melatonin is power anti-stress and anticancer hormone.

Yoga Nidra

It is divine sleep with alertness. In 15 minute yoga nidra session, you relax in a fully supported shavasan, limbs limp, breath quiet, thoughts drifting by. In the distance, the 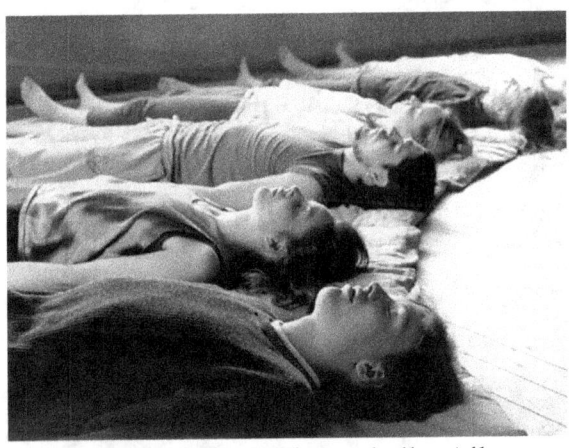 teacher's voice blends with the sound of Tibetan bells. All traces of the day fade away, time stops, and stillness washes over the body. Yoga nidra is a systematic method of complete relaxation, holistically addressing our physiological, neurological, and subconscious needs.

How long should you take this protocol?

If all is well patient feels better and tumor start to shrink within a 3 or 4 months, if he follows treatment religiously and honestly. He may be cured in one or two years. **It is recommended that the Budwig protocol and full diet is followed for at least five years.** Even after that he should maintain healthy eating and life style.

Dr. Budwig has clearly mentioned that if you do not get the desired success, do not blame the protocol, rather try to find out your mistakes and correct them. The threshold between winning and losing is very small, and even a minor mistake can unbalance the complete healing process.

How do I recognize a good Flax seed oil?

Good Flax seed oil is unfortunately dependent on many factors. The IOPDF assigns a star for each fulfilled criterion. The best oil has thus 6 stars and the worst gets no star. Let us look at the 6 criteria in detail:

Criterion 1: Cooling chain

Studies have shown that, in addition to processing the Flax seed, cooling is the most important criterion for a good Flax seed oil. So buy only Flax seed oil stored in a refrigerated rack and kept in a permanent cold chain. If you shop through the Internet, the Flax seed oil must be delivered in a Styrofoam packaging and as fast as possible.

Criterion 2: Local Flax seed

Weekly shipping on ships and sometimes additional chemicals used can cause great damage to Flax seed. Therefore, make sure that you only buy Flax seed oil whose Flax seed comes from the country where you are living or at least from the same continent. This normally can be seen at the seal.

Criterion 3: Omega-3 fatty acid content

The Oil-Protein Diet is about linolenic acid (omega-3). Buy Flax seed oil with a high amount of linolenic acid. Depending in which country you are living the range can be between 55% - 63%.

Criterion 4: Organic quality

It makes a big difference whether Flax seed grows in biologically controlled soil or in soils of conventional agriculture. So buy only Flax seed oils with organic quality, unless you know the oil mill personally and know what Flax seed the mill is processing.

Criterion 5: glass bottle

Flax seed oil and electron differentiation oils are available in glass and plastic bottles or in canisters, which are mostly made of tinplate. Consumers should only buy oils in glass bottles. Avoid plastic bottles, as they may contain highly toxic softeners.

Criterion 6: Light

Flax seed oil should be packaged and stored in a light-proof package. Therefore, only buy bottles in dark brown or dark green bottles. (Oil Protein Diet by Lothar Hieneise)

Linomel

Linomel is an invention by Dr Budwig. Freshly crushed Flax seed is mixed with honey and milk powder so that the crushed Flax seed is more stable. There is no doubt that freshly crushed Flax seed is more valuable, but also has the disadvantage that you do it yourself and clean the grinder afterwards. That is why Linomel still has an existence right. Do not buy crushed Flax seed in the shop as the chance that these contain Trans fatty acids is 100%.

Is there an alternative to Linomel?

- Freshly crushed Flax seed is an alternative. This must be eaten immediately after the meal, otherwise it will oxidize.
- Make your own Linomel. Mix 6 tablespoons freshly crushed Flax seed with a tablespoon of honey. Small tip: Grind the Flax seed, e.g. in a coffee grinder, and set the grinder to coarse. So it mixes better with the honey.

(Oil Protein Diet by Lothar Hieneise)

Questions and Answers

How do I store Flax seed oil?

Generally cool. Best at 5^0-10^0 (Fahrenheit 41-50) in the refrigerator. Always keep the Flax seed oil bottles upright and never lay them down as they may cause faster oxidation.

Should I now buy low fat Quark or Quark with 20% or 40% fat?

Only a Quark with as little fat (less than 2%) is optimal. Quark is about sulfur-containing amino acids. Less fat means more amino acids.

Can Quark be replaced with tofu, yoghurt or soya?

Absolutely no.

Is there an alternative to Quark?

In many books or on the Internet, it is always claimed that there are alternatives to Quark, such as e.g., yogurt, soy or whey protein (which you should never use!). This is wrong. There is absolutely no good substitute for Quark. The only alternative (although it has a slightly different composition like Quark) is Cottage Cheesewith as little fat as possible. This should only be used if no Quark is available.

Can I eat cheese?

Basically yes, but in moderation and with the exception of cream cheese and fresh cheese. Only raw milk/hard cheese is permitted. Cheese of sheep or goat is preferable.

Can I eat raisins and dates?

Yes, raisins and dates are allowed in small quantities.

Which fat can be used for frying?

Only coconut fat.

Can I use olive oil?

Theoretically, you can use any organic oils with salad. Dr Budwig preferred Flax seed oil, pumpkin seed oil, wheat germ oil, poppy oil, and thistle oil are also permitted, but do not heat. Oleolox may be heated for two minutes.

Can I drink coffee?

No.

Can soya and oatmeal be eaten?

Dr Budwig wrote several times that oat flakes, soy flakes, yeast flakes and other flakes are permitted. But today I just say that you buy only high quality organic "flakes".

Can I eat bread?

Dr Budwig has recommended her patients to eat no bread during acute tumor phases. Instead, she recommended full-grain rice waffles or Ezekiel bread as an alternative.

Can cows or soy milk be drunk?

No, drinking any milk is forbidden in the Oil-Protein Diet.

Can noodles be eaten?

In the literature of Dr Budwig nearly always did not allow cancer patients to eat noodles. The reason is that noodles are made of flour, eggs and oil. Flour has the disadvantage that it is basically a fast-digesting sugar and mostly the producers use cheap oils. Energetically speaking, noodles are "not really full with electrons". Unfortunately, you are worsening the already bad adrenaline - insulin ratio of a cancer patient.

Which milk can be used for the Quark?

Dr Budwig recommended raw milk. Unfortunately these are nowadays difficult to buy anywhere. Alternatively, pasteurized milk is also okay. All other varieties of milk, such as ultra-heat-treated or homogenized (long life or full cream), are prohibited.

Budwig Diet & Protocol - In Brief

This is raw organic diet with lot of Flax oil and Juices. Consume only clean or RO filtered water. To get the best results, proper guidance is strongly recommended. Below are brief guidelines of the Budwig Diet you don't have to consume all the foods on this list. This information is from Dr. Budwig's books.

First thing in the morning – One glass of sauerkraut juice, preferably raw & homemade. Raw unheated kraut has enzymes, probiotics and vitamins which help the digestive system, metabolize foods & improve immunity.

Just before breakfast - green or herbal tea

Breakfast – First blend 3 Tbsp. Flax oil, 3 Tbsp. milk and a Tsp real honey; then gradually add 6 Tbsp. Quark or Cottage Cheeseand blend. Garnish in layers. Add 2 Tbsp freshly ground Flax seeds n a bowl, then add a layer of crushed fresh fruits, then pour oil cheese mixture and put raw nuts on top. Afterward, if hungry, choose whole grain organic bread, raw vegetables, & quality cheeses such as Edam, Gouda, Emmentaler, Sbrinz or Camembert.

Mid-morning - Homemade vegetable juice (carrots, beets w/lemon or apple, or greens). Homemade carrot or beet juices are very important cancer-fighters.

Before Lunch (especially serious patients) - Champagne with 1 Tbsp ground Flax seeds in small glass of fruit juice. The champagne helps with absorption of the seeds.

Lunch - Salad plate (tomato, cucumber, lettuce, radish, cabbage, broccoli, and pepper) with homemade Cottage Cheeseand Flax oil mayo dressing (prepared by mixing together 2 Tbsp Flax oil, 2 Tbsp milk, 2 Tbsp Cottage Cheeseand 1 Tbsp lemon juice, add a variety of herbs making the plate most appealing.

Lunch - Main Course Vegetables cooked in water, then flavored with oleolox and herbs possibly with oatmeal, curry etc. Vegetable soups flavored with a little oleolux and nutritional yeast flakes, as side dish for buckwheat, brown rice, millet or potatoes.

Lunch Dessert - Must have 2nd serving of 3 Tbsp. Flax oil and 6 Tbsp. Quark or Cottage Cheesewith a little milk and honey, well blended. Add raw fruit, fruit juice, raw nuts, and other flavors you like.

Mid-afternoon - 1 Tbsp. freshly ground Flax seed added to 1 glass of pure fruit juice, homemade.

Late afternoon - Papaya or pineapple juice, 1 glass, with 1 Tbsp Flax seeds freshly ground.

Dinner - Grains alone or grains & beans with vegetables with oleolox, nutritional yeast flakes & spices. Eat buckwheat at least 4 days in a week. Grains & beans combined make a complete protein. Vegetables such as spinach, asparagus, broccoli, & cabbage add nutrition and aid absorption. Dine early.

Late Evening - 1 glass red wine (optional). Go to sleep early - before 10 P.M. if possible.

Prohibitions of Budwig Protocol
- No Sugar, no meat, no eggs, no Butter
- No hydrogenated fat and refined oil
- No soya, corn, peanuts and refined table salt
- No frying, no sautéing, no deep frying
- No preservatives and processed Food
- No microwave, teflon coated and aluminum cookware
- No cosmetics, chemicals and pesticides
- No foam mattress and pillow.
- No nylon, polyester or acrylic clothing, only cotton, silk and wool is allowed.
- No Crt. TV and mobile phones
- No leftover food

Elimination or Detoxification
May include (Remember the Mnemonic - M.Sc. Botany)

- **Flax oil massage,**
- **sun therapy,**
- **coffee enema** and
- **soda bicarb bath,** epsom bath, oil pulling, steam bath, sauna bath, liver, colon and kidney cleansing etc.

Energy Therapies (Remember MTV)

- **Meditation**, Meditation, yoga nidra, positive attitude, system change and deep breathing exercises.
- **Tumor contract** – Tell your tumor that if it grows in size, then you may die, and eventually he also will die. So advise him to become microscopic in size. In return you promise to make some changes in your life so that both of you might live long. If he agrees with your proposal, sign a contract with him immediately.
- **Visualization** – is the most important tool to tap into the power of your imagination to help heal cancer. Remain tuned to your healthy and happy future.

Important and must do therapies with Budwig

- Dandelion root 1 Tsp once or twice a day
- Black seed oil as advised by Maria Hurairah
- Bitter apricot kernels 5 kernels per 5kg of body weight with a Tsp pumpkin seeds
- Essiac tea 30ml to 90ml per day
- Brazil nuts a nut a day
- Nano curcumin 1 cap twice or thrice a day
- and Coenyme Q-10 1 cap once or twice a day
- Nutritional yeast flakes

Lothar Hirneise

Great supporter of Budwig Protocol

Eleven years, Lothar Hirneise worked as a trained nurse in the State Psychiatric Hospital in Winnenden. After four years, he took psychoanalysis training. Hirneise was also master in Eastern combat sports and a Kung Fu teacher. He owned a successful sporting goods company, which he sold for a tidy profit in 1986. After a year one of his close friend developed Testicular Cancer. Lothar went in search of information about 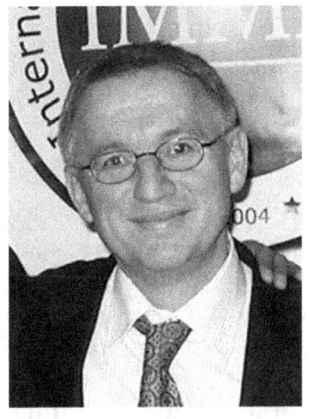 cancer therapies and came across Lynne McTaggart, the founder of the book and magazine "What Doctor's Don't Tell You." Then he was informed that Frank Wiewel, president of the American organization "People Against Cancer", which operates alternative cancer research since 1985, would come to London. So he went to London with his best friend Klaus Pertl to attend this conference for alternative cancer treatments (early 1997). This weekend his friend died. This was the starting point of his intensive quest for potential cancer therapies. He had time and money and read everything he could get his hands on. He nearly went crazy and was severely infected by a virus called Holistic Oncology. He travelled to Bahamas, Mexico, Russia, China, and the United States and all over Europe.

Frank Wiewel advised him to visit Dr. Budwig who lived only 60 km from his home in Germany. Lothar and Klaus Pertl visited Budwig in the spring of 1998, and from the beginning it was an intense relationship that persisted for a very long time.

Over several years he remained in close contact with this great sage of Science. The content of their conversations used to be about fats and electrons. One day she suggested writing a book in which, she could explain her theories again, briefly and concisely. And the Book Cancer - "The Problem And The Solution" was written. Lothar worked very hard in the creation of this great book.

Lothar Hirneise is founder and President of "People Against Cancer", Germany. He is a great researcher and writer on alternative healing. In his book "Chemotherapy cures cancer and the earth is flat" he puts an "Encyclopedia of unconventional cancer treatments", and summarizes the results of his years of worldwide research together. The book became a best seller within no time. He had successfully treated thousands of cancer patients at his center in Germany (3E Zentrum, Buocher Höhe Im Salenhäule 10, D-73630 Remshalden-Buoch Telefon: 07151-98130).

Tumor is not a problem, but a solution

Lothar Hirneise says: "A tumor is the body's solution to some problem in your body. A tumor forms because someone is no longer producing adrenaline, which is needed to break down sugar. An excess of sugar is dangerous, so the body produces tumors. Tumors ferment or burn sugar. Tumors also use a lot of energy - sugar - due to the fast division of cells. Cancer cells function like liver cells, but much more efficiently. So the tumor helps you to get rid of poisons from your body. Without the tumor you would be really ill. That is why you shouldn't immediately operate to remove a tumor. First strengthen and detoxify yourself. If the tumor still continues to grow - which is almost never the case - you can always operate later."

3E Program

He travels a lot in search of finding most successful alternative cancer therapies. In the last few years he has interviewed several hundred final stage so-called survivors, meaning patients who were in the final stage of cancer and who are all healthy again today. Based on his findings he proposed a 3E Program for cancer.

- Eat well
- Eliminate the toxins from the body
- Energy

He noticed that 100% of all survivors, did the energy work. In approximately - say 80% of all patients, He found a change in diet. And in at least 60% of all patients, took intensive detoxification rituals. This is the basis of his, so much talked about 3E Program for healing cancer.

Diet and Nutrition

He proudly says that he has shaken the hands with hundreds of people, who made extreme dietary change and became well. They are still alive and living a healthy life. If you still believe that Cancer diets are nonsense, go to him, he will prove the opposite. He has interviewed enough patients and knows them personally. Good nutrition naturally means getting energy. He explains that we have three ways and means of getting energy into our bodies.

1. The first is the light. Light is naturally our number one source of energy. He is 100% sure.

2. The second way is organic nutrition. He emphasized strict organic diet; of course, you do not get any energy from a chicken burger. Rather, when you eat this, you lose some energy, which you have to compensate later.

3. Another possibility which you have is let the energy flow in your body, in your meridians and in your thoughts. Think

about the feeling you had last time when you were in love. You felt wonderful; you were on top of the sky. But what did it change? Did your DNA change? Did your cell respiration change? Nothing really changed. The Indians would say your chakras were opened and the energy started to flow freely again. This is the secret, not only to get the energy, but also to let it flow freely. This proves that our thoughts, our mental-spiritual side is too important.

Now back to nutrition. Out of all nutritional therapies of cancer that he had investigated, the Budwig diet is definitely number one. He investigated thousands of patients, Dr. Budwig allowed him to investigate all her cases of the last thirty years, and he concluded that nowhere you find such fantastic cases as with Dr. Budwig, not even remotely. It's amazing. Even patients who were in coma, when received her Oil-Protein Diet, and rubbed so-called electron differential oils (ELDI oils) on the body, did again come out from coma. They were able to eat, walk and live normally today. It is really miraculous. Therefore, her Oil-Protein Diet became the basis of his 3-E Program for cancer patients.

Detoxification

Next important point that he suggests is detoxification. Detoxification actually covers two points.

1. The first is naturally to avoid toxins and poisons e.g. use of cosmetics, toothpaste, etc.

2. And the second point which belongs to detoxification is not to add any toxins in future. The most important point is definitely diet. It doesn't need further explanation. We are ingesting lot of poisons through our diet. Is better not to eat than all this rubbish that one can buy today.

Healthy teeth and gums are phenomenally important. Heat is a very good way to expel poisons. All the parasite cleanses, colon cleansing, ELDI oils, drinking a lot of water is essential. Going out into the sun light, twice daily is very important. You might

108

have listened today that the sun is suddenly bad for you and may cause skin cancer. That is nonsense, forget it. We are all children of the light, we definitely need the light. Even if it's raining and cloudy today go outside. Even if patient is in coma, he must be wheeled out. You should go twice daily into the light. Light increases Vitamin D levels, important for the liver and increases energy levels.

Energy Work

Energy work is the most important point. He divides it into mental and spiritual work. Naturally, you are advised to do meditation and develop positive thinking. You think about life, 'Why do I have cancer and what is the purpose of my life, why am I here on this earth?' and so on. But he focused on something what he called the **SYSTEM CHANGE**. He explains that we all live in Systems. In our marriage, in our house, in our job, etc. Many, many, many of these cancer patients made system jumps. Means that they kicked their husband in the butt and threw him out. They quit their job, they moved, they not only moved their bed, they moved out of their apartment, went to other countries. Quite honestly, I don't know, what should you do? But Lother's experience is that it it's remarkable to what extent people changed their life before they were in a position to get well.

Lothar Hirneise Concludes: "There is no spontaneous remission, there are only people who positively change their life and regained their health that way." (Hirneise, 2005)

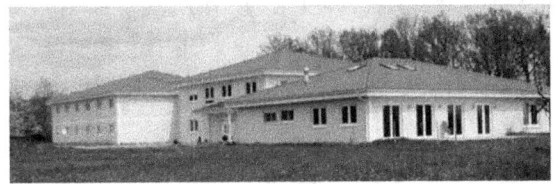

~~.**~~

109

Interview of Dr. Johanna Budwig

Lothar Hirneise worked with Dr. Johanna Budwig from 1998 to 2003. He explained that there is much more available to cancer patients than just chemo and irradiation. Mr. Lothar Hirneise conducted this great interview in 1998 (Budwig, Cancer The Problem And The Solution).

Lothar Hirneise: What is your fundamental research?

Dr Johanna Budwig: In 1949, I developed Paper Chromatography of fats with Professor Kaufmann, the director of the Federal Institute for Research on Grain, Potatoes and Fat, and my former doctoral advisor, who was also director of the Pharmaceutical Institute. With this technique for first time I was able to detect fats, fatty acids and lipoproteins directly even in 0.1 ml of blood. I used Co 60 isotopes successfully to produce the first differential reaction for fatty 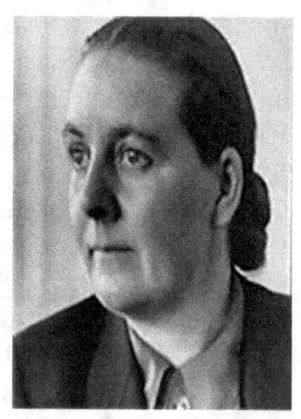 acids, and produced the first direct iodine value via radioiodine. I also developed control of atmosphere in closed system by using gas systems which act as antioxidants. I further developed Coloring, separating effects of fats and fatty acids. I too studied their behavior in blue light, red light with fluorescent dyes.

Using rhodamine red dye, I studied the electrical behavior of the unsaturated fatty acids with their "halo". With this technique I could prove that electron rich highly unsaturated Linoleic and Linolenic fatty acids (Flax oil being richest source) were the mysterious and undiscovered decisive fats in respiratory enzyme function which Otto Warburg could not find. I studied the electromagnetic function of pi-electrons of the linolenic acid in the cell membranes, for all nerve function, secretions, mitosis, as

110

well as cell division. I also examined the synergism of the sulfur containing protein with the Pi-electrons of the highly unsaturated fatty acids and their significance for the formation of the hydrogen bridge between fat and protein, which represent "the only path" for fast and focused Transport of electrons during respiration.

This immediately caused an excitement in scientific community. Everybody thought that it will open new doors in Cancer research. I also proved that Hydrogenated fats, refined oils including all Trans fatty acids were not having any vital electrons and thus proved as respiratory poisons. We published this research exclusively in many journals including "New Directions in Fat Research".

Lothar Hirneise: What is the prime cause of Cancer?

Dr Johanna Budwig: In 1928 Dr. Otto Warburg proved that all normal cells require oxygen absolutely, but cancer cells can live without oxygen. It is a rule without exception. If you deprive a cell 35% of its oxygen for 48 hours and it would become cancerous. Dr. Otto Warburg has proved it clearly that the root cause of cancer is lack of oxygen in the cells, which creates an acidic state in the human body.

He also discovered that cancer cells are anaerobic i.e. do not breathe oxygen, get the energy by fermentation of glucose producing lactic acid and cannot thrive in the presence of high levels of oxygen. Long back in 1911 Swedish scientist Torsten Thunberg postulated that sulfur containing protein (found in cottage cheese) and some unknown fat is required to attract oxygen in the cell. This fat plays a major role in the cellular respiration. For nearly half century scientists were trying to identify this unknown and mysterious fat but nobody succeeded.

Lothar Hirneise: How did you develop cancer therapy which is called Budwig Protocol?

Dr Johanna Budwig: During my research I found that the blood of seriously ill cancer patients had deficiency of unsaturated essential fats (Linoleic and Linolenic fatty acids),

111

lipoproteins, phosphatides, and hemoglobin. I also noticed that cancer patients had a strange greenish-yellow substance in their blood which is not present in the blood of healthy people. I wanted to develop a healing program for cancer.

So I decided to straight way go for human trials and I enrolled 642 cancer patients from four big hospitals in Münster. I started to give Flax oil and Cottage Cheeseto the cancer patients. After just three months, patients began to improve in health and strength, the yellow green substance in their blood began to disappear, tumors gradually receded and at the same time as the nutrients began to rise. Thus I had a cure for cancer. It was a great victory and the first milestone in the battle against cancer. My treatment is based on the consumption of Flax seed oil with low fat cottage cheese, raw organic diet, detoxification, mild exercise, Flax oil massage and the healing powers of the sun. I have treated approx. 2500 cancer patients during last few decades. Prof. Halme of surgery clinic in Helsinki used to keep records of my patients. According to him my success was over 90% and this too was achieved in cases where conventional Oncology failed.

Lothar Hirneise: Can you tell us more about the unsaturated fatty acids and their net-like connections?

Dr. Johanna Budwig: Fatty acid is a carboxylic acid having unbranched chain of 4 to 28 carbons. The saturated fatty acids have primarily short carbon chains. In butter, coconut fat, goat fat and sheep fat the fatty acids consists of 4, 6, 8, 10 or 12 carbons. These fats are saturated, however they can also easily metabolize if the essential fatty acids are present. The unsaturated vital fatty acids really start with the chain with 18 carbon compounds. There are also fatty acids with up to 30 carbons. Fatty acids with 18 carbons, like in Flax oil with the higher level of unsaturation, are more important for human beings, particularly for the brain functions of man. Linoleic acid rich in electrons is considered vital. There is particularly high amount of energy in this double double bonds of the linoleic acid.

112

This energy wanders and is not fixed in place while in a chemical compound, such as with table salt the energy is fixed. This energy, wandering between electrons and the positively charged protein with sulfur groups is an alternating association process in the electromagnetic field. This is very important. Perhaps you are familiar with the painting of Michelangelo, where God creates Adam (two fingers pointing to each other, however they do not touch). This is quantum physics, here the fingers do not touch. The physicists who I know, Max Planck, or Albert Einstein, or Dessauer all represent the view that man is created by God in His image. You see in being together as human beings there is certainly also a connection without directly touching the other person. The dipolarity with a single double bond in olive oil is weaker than it is in sunflower seed oil, which is has two double bonds. This double double bond is considered to be vital for man. However if the same chain length of 18 carbons has three unsaturated fatty acid double bonds, then the electrical energy is as strong as a magnet. This electronic energy is negatively charged. The positively charged sulfur groups of the protein adhere in the unsaturated bonds where the electrons are and that is where they insert their sulfur-containing compounds.

This produces the lipoproteins. The life process is sustained in the interplay between the positively-charged particles and negatively-charged particles. In this process there is no connection, and this is our life element. If radical damage occurs at this point through fatty acids that has lost electron energy, but rather are cross-linked like a net, then the dipolarity can no longer work actively in this net. This is the deadly effect of free radicals, because instead of the chains with the electron clouds they interlace like a net without electron clouds, indeed with unsaturated bonds, but without dipolarity. I quickly knew that the triple unsaturated fatty acids, which were called linolenic acid, and which no one had isolated before me, had 18 carbons and that they did not always carry their double bonds at the same point. They have such a strong electronic energy compared to the heavier matter in the 18-link fatty acid chains, that biologically

113

this energy is far greater than it is with the next arachidonic acid with 20 links. The highest electron collection is with the combination of linoleic-linolenic fatty acids in Flax oil. The linolenic acid as conjugated (interaction of neighboring double bonds in the molecule that are separated by a single bond) fatty acid is even more effective and is even more strongly interplay with linoleic acid as it is present in the Flax oil for oxygen absorption. This was relatively easy for me to verify in my experiments. I would like to emphasize this. The combination of double unsaturated linoleic acid with triple unsaturated linolenic acid is particularly well-combined in Flax seed.

Lothar Hirneise: Is it this energy that heals cancer?

Dr. Johanna Budwig: Yes, this energy is now movable and it is easily released. It is precisely this energy that heals cancer, or does not even allow it to occur. If this vital element is present then no tumor can exist. This vital element is a deciding factor in the immune system. There is no effective factor in the immune system other than the essential fatty acids.

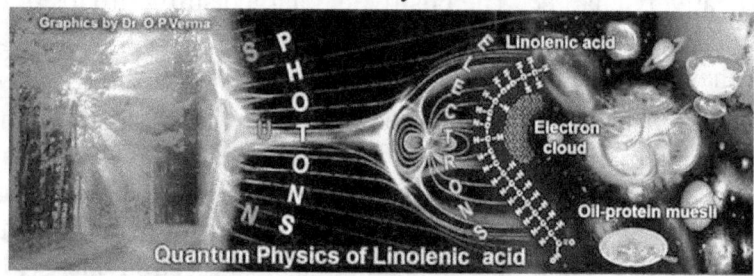

Lothar Hirneise: What is an electron cloud?

Dr Johanna Budwig: If the enhancement of electronic energy is always higher through absorption of sun photons in the unsaturated fatty acids e.g. in linolenic fatty acids, then the power of the electrons is so high in the dipolarity between gravity and electrons, that they lifts off of the heavy mass and floats like a cloud hence I called them electron cloud.

Lothar Hirneise: What is the significance of the cloud?

Dr. Johanna Budwig: No life form has as much energy to store the electrons and photons as doe's man. The electronic

114

energy stored particularly in the vital, highly unsaturated fatty acids, is very strong life element for man. Man cannot live without them. If oils are treated with heat and harsh chemicals (during refining and hydrogenation process to increase their shelf life) then the wealth of vital electronic energy is destroyed and Trans fats are formed with net like connections. They are no longer vital fats with 18 carbons, but rather they form cross-links between the fatty acids like a large net, and are highly damaging to our body, do not adhere with proteins, do not attract oxygen and act like a free radicals. I repeat because it is so important: I have detected particles in oils treated with steam, which indeed have a positive iodine value, but which are highly toxic for man.

Lothar Hirneise: So you preach against these toxic hydrogenated and refined oils?

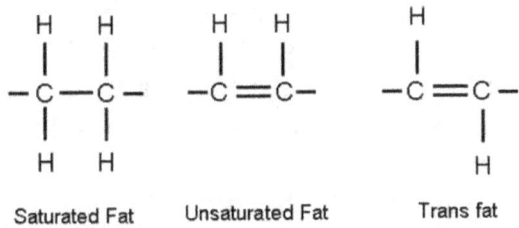

Saturated Fat   Unsaturated Fat   Trans fat

Dr. Johanna Budwig: I am completely against using these "pseudo" fats - "hydrogenated" or "partially hydrogenated". These are the biggest enemy of mankind. I had scientific proofs. The heart rejects these fats and they are deposited as inorganic fat on the heart muscle itself. They end up blocking circulation, damage heart action, inhibit cell renewal and impede the free flow of blood and lymph fluids.

But it was highly profitable business for multinationals. When I preached against these fats, they stood against me, first they tried to bribe me and when I refused they filed many fake court cases against me. I was working for humanity and had scientific proof. I was like rock of Gibraltar in my decision; I fought and won all the cases ultimately.

Lothar Hirneise: What is your view point about surgery for tumors?

Dr. Johanna Budwig: I am totally against radiation and chemo; I also reject hormonal treatment. Surgery must be considered individually. I am not a proponent of quickly making artificial anus. Conventional oncology no longer does justice to the cancer patients.

Lothar Hirneise: You also studied medicine at the age of 47 years.

Dr. Johanna Budwig: (smiling) Yes handsome! That's right, my opponents were accusing me that how can I treat cancer patients without a doctors degree. This thing pinched me, so in 1955, I joined medical school in Göttingen. There I was using my therapy very successfully in various clinics. I still remember the time I was working late one night in Göttingen, a woman came to me, with her small child whose arm was supposed to be amputated due to a tumor. I treated her and soon the subject of amputation was dismissed and the child quickly did very well.

Because I was still a medical student at this time, I was summoned to appear before the Municipal Court due to a petition that I should be prohibited from studying medicine. I explained the truth in the court. The judge rejected the case and said, "You have done a good job, Budwig. In my area of jurisdiction nothing will happen to you. If it does there will be a scandal in the scientific community."

Lothar Hirneise: What do you recommend for prevention of cancer?

Dr. Johanna Budwig: Consume only Flax oil as oil. I reject frozen and preserved meat. Fresh meat is OK. No frozen food and no bakery products. No Trans fats. Eat organic diet. Oleolox should be used as butter. Prepare fruit juices yourself. Cheese and potatoes are OK. Also the electromagnetic environment (e.g. microwave and mobile phones etc.) in which we live is very important. I reject synthetic textiles and foam mattresses because

116

they steal lot of electrons from you. A lot of wood in home construction and woolen or silk carpets are also important. Wear gemstones, they also have good biological radiation. Books could be written on gemstones. The environment and living conditions must be as biological (organic & natural) as possible. Regular sleep is very important.

Sun, Photons and Electrons

Sun, photons, electrons - What are they?

Sun rays reach the earth as an inexhaustible source of energy. The sources of power in mineral oil, coal, green plant-foods and fruits are based on the energy supplied by the sun's radiation. Light is the fastest traveler from star to star. There is nothing that travels faster than light. Light speeds along with time. Physicists emphasize that the photon, the quantum, the smallest component of the sun's rays is eternal. It is truly a life element. Life is impossible without the photon.

The photon is always in motion. Nothing can ever halt its motion. The photon is full of colors and can change its color, its frequency, when present in large numbers. The photon - acknowledged to be the purest form of energy, the purest wave, always in motion—can unite with a second photon, when it is in resonance with the other, to form a "short-lived particle." This particle, known as "O" particle, can break up into two photons again, without mass, as a pure wave in motion. This is the basis for the wonderful back and forth movement between light and matter. This photon can never be pinned down to one location. This is the foundation for the Theory of Relativity. The photon gave rise to Max Planck's and Einstein's formation of the quantum theory which is of such significance today.

Electrons

Electrons are a smallest particles of matter and are in continual movements. They vibrate continually on their own wavelength. They have their own frequency, like radio receivers which are set at a certain wavelength. The electron orbits in matter around a nucleus. The heavy matter in the nucleus (proton) is charged with positive electricity. In contrast to this, the electron carries a negative charge. The positively charged nucleus and the negatively charged electron attract each other by

118

means of their electrical opposition. But the electron, always in motion, never approaches the nucleus close enough to be drawn out of its own orbit. It maintains a certain freedom of movement within its prescribed orbit.

The electron loves photons. It attracts photons by its magnetic field. When an electrical charge moves, it always produces a magnetic field. The moving photon also has a magnetic field. Both fields, the magnetic field of the electrons and the magnetic field of the photons attract each other when the wavelengths are in tune. The wave length of the photon—which the photon can change—must fit into the wavelength of the orbiting electron so that the orbit maintains a complete wavelength. This feature is extremely interesting in terms of its physical, biological and even philosophical consequences. Matter always has its own vibration, and so, of course, does the living body. The absorption of energy must correspond to one's own wavelength.

Sunbeams are very much in harmony with human. It is no coincidence that we love the sun. The quantum biologists say that the resonance in our body is so strongly tuned to the sun's energy that: There is nothing else on earth with a higher concentration of photons of the sun's energy than man. This concentration of the sun's energy with their highly suitable wavelengths is improved when we eat electron-rich food. The electrons attract the electromagnetic waves of sunbeams. Flax seed oil contain high amount of electrons which are on the wavelength of the sun's energy. Scientifically, these oils are even known as electron-rich essential highly unsaturated fats. *The famous Quantum Physicist Dessauer writes: If it were possible to increase' the concentration of solar electrons tenfold in this electron-rich unsaturated fats, then man would be able to live 10,000 years.*

The sun's energy and man as an antenna

Almost everyone knows what an antenna is. The marvelous science of Maxwell, the physicist, concerning electro-magnetic waves today are well-researched and of practical use. Famous examples are telegraphy, radio, television, microwave oven, cell phones and various applications of high-frequency technology in the manufacturing of electromagnets, the atom bomb and research into nuclear power as a source of energy. Maxwell was able to show that an electric current flowing in an electrically conductive matter produces a magnetic field. Also electrically conductive matter which is moved within a magnet's field, will produce a current. When an atomic particle, such as an electron, is accelerated by an electric field, this produces electric and magnetic fields, which travel at right angles to each other, produces electromagnetic wave. These fundamental, elementary laws can also be applied to biological processes.

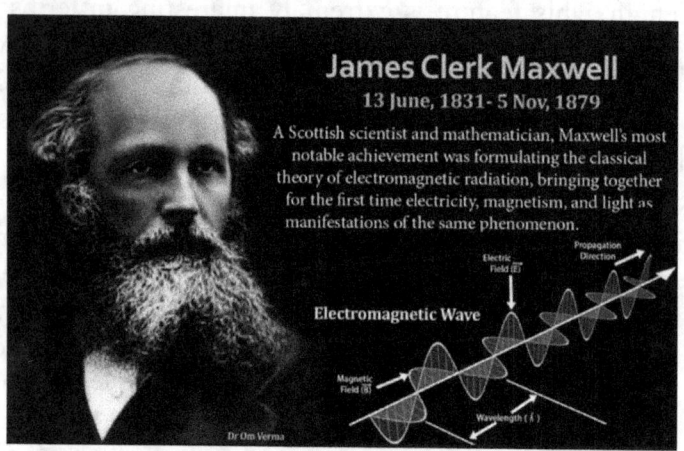

When the sun shines on the leafy canopy of a tree and is absorbed through photosynthesis, this causes movement in the electrical charge of the electrons. A magnetic field is also brought about when the water in trees rises. When we, with our wealth of electrons and conductive living substance, move through the electro-magnetic field of a forest, then a charging with solar electrons takes place in us. When our blood circulates, there is a movement of the electrical charge in the magnetic fields (for example, on the surface lipids of red blood corpuscles), which then causes much induction and re-induction of energy.

With each heartbeat, a dose of the body's own electron-rich, highly unsaturated fats from the lymph system, together with lymph fluid, goes into the blood vessels and thereby into the heart. This constantly stimulates and strengthens the electro-motoric functioning of the heart; Even the movement of the bloodstream is connected with radiation of electromagnetic waves-in accordance with the fundamental law of nature which governs electro-magnetic waves. This Transmitter within humans is always in action.

This Transmitter is also observed in neurons. The cylindrical structure of our nerves with the different layers and ganglions, with the difference in electrical potential between the neurons and dendrites, immediately supplies the picture of how strongly an electric current in a magnetic field leads to the emitting of electromagnetic waves. When I think a positive thought about another person, this involves the emitting of electromagnetic waves. The reception of thought also depends on the wavelength to which the receiver is tuned. There are amplifiers, as well as Transmitters that interfere. This encompasses a whole host of situations that are known under different names such as telepathy, hypnosis, mental telepathy, and many others.

Among Nordic peoples, it is known that the isolated native inhabitants use a tree to amplify thought Transmission, for example, to inform the husband who had gone to town, that he should bring back some salt. Bismark described how, during periods of trouble or pressure, he found relaxation by putting his arms around a tree and leaning his forehead against the trunk. In both cases, it involves electromagnetic waves that behave in accord with Maxwell's mathematical equations.

Fats Syndrome

The special relationship between photons, electrons and Essential Fats (EFAs) described by Dr. Budwig is due to the amazing molecular structures of LA (cis-linoleic acid) and ALA (cis-linolenic acid). The cis-configuration allows de-localized electron clouds (pi-electrons) to collect in the bend produced on the chain. The resulting electrostatic force enables the EFAs to capture oxygen molecules and hold proteins within cell membranes. Like static electricity in a capacitor these charges can produce measurable bioelectric currents essential to nerve, muscle, heart and membrane functions. EFAs are extremely important to the body's overall energy exchange potential — the flow of life force.

Let us concentrate on the actual fats syndrome with its effects on the brain and nerve functions, the organs of the senses, the secretion of mucous, the functioning of the stomach and intestinal tract, liver, gall bladder and kidneys, the lymph and blood vessels, the skin, respiration, the immunity system, the fertilization processes and sexuality. All of these systems and processes of the human being are very much connected with electron-rich highly unsaturated fats, as receivers, amplifiers and Transmitters of electro-magnetic waves, and as supervisor of the vital functions. *The famous Quantum Physicist Dessauer writes: If it were possible to increase the concentration of solar electrons tenfold in this electron-rich unsaturated fat molecule, then man would be able to live 10,000 years.*

Anti-Mensch

Physicists interpret from mathematical formulae that man, with his wealth of electrons, is directed forward in time, which conceals within him the greatest potential to attract the sun's energy, and is directed against entropy. By means of these mathematical formulae, applied to Physics, and by reversing time, the mirror image of human beings is coined—the "Anti-Mensch", lacking electrons, lacks power and strength and directed into the past. It increases the occurrence of cancer. His thought processes, too—is paralyzed, because the element of life, the sun-attuned electrons, is missing.

The process by which x-rays, gamma rays, atom bombs or cobalt rays are set in motion is also equally directed toward the development of the "Anti-Mensch". The electronic structure of the vital functions is destroyed by such rays. According to Feynman's "World Line Diagram" and modern theory of relativity, time and space have been given a relationship in a formula. The "Anti-Mensch" is directed into the past. Human's body tissues with its interplay between solar energy photons and large number of electrons, with its concentration of photons in life's activities and in the dynamics of the vital functions, are directed into the future.

But, when people began to hydrogenate the oils to increase their shelf-life; no-one thought about the consequences of this. In this process these vitally important electrons were destroyed. During hydrogenation, vegetable oils are reacted with hydrogen gas at high temperature. A nickel is used to speed up the reaction and unsaturated fats are hardened. This negative aspect concerning the development of the "Anti-Mensch" is in accordance with Feynman's "World Line Diagram". I emphasize that it means the fats and oils which have had their electron structure destroyed serve, within time and space, to promote the development of the "Anti-Mensch".

The electrons as resonance system

The electrons in our food serve as the resonance system for the sun's energy. Their electro-magnetic field attracts the photons in sunlight. The physicist cannot imagine life without these active and vital photons. These photons, which are in resonance with the electrons in seed oils, are focused on the same wavelength as the sun's energy, serve the life element. This interplay of solar energy photons and the electrons in seed oils governs all the vital functions. Fats are the dominant factor for all the vital functions, according to Ivar Bang.

The electrons of highly unsaturated fats from seed oils, which are on the same wavelength as sunlight, are capable of drawing solar energy and storing it, then, upon demand, of activating it as the purest energy in the form of the electrons clouds, and making it available for the vital functions. All the vital functions are closely connected with membrane function.

The exchange of electrons, the distribution of energy in the whole organism is dependent on these membrane functions — in the nerve pathways, the brain, in every organ, the liver, gall bladder and pancreas in the stomach's mucous membrane and in the kidneys and intestinal tract. The controlling functions of these membranes with their electro-motoric power, is felt everywhere. This is also true for the respiratory functions, and in oxygen absorption and utilization. It also applies to cell division — to all normal growth processes. It is true for the catabolism of substance in the elimination processes taking place by way of the kidneys, intestinal tract and also for the growth of hair and nails, as well as for the development of young life in the womb. Most significant point is that it is this electronic energy that heals cancer. This turning point in the field of proven successful cancer therapy is only one aspect of much bigger picture of the Quantum Biology. A lot of mysteries and miracles have yet to be discovered by doing research in Quantum Biology.

How can we once more reach the peak of human development?

Freeing you from the influences and effects of radiation and from environmental factors which promote development into the "Anti-Mensch", seem important. These goals, set by the individual who chooses, or by the state and food industries with their organization and planning, should be to see that the food we eat consists of electron-rich nutrition. An electron-rich food intake which supplies us with the resonance system for the sun's energy, must once more achieve priority. Such food, as the life element, promotes our sun-attuned energy. This in turn promotes our development, in space and time, into the future. The entire self can then grow and continue to develop further until, in accordance with the laws of nature which govern light and life, the highest level of our being is achieved. *(Excerpted from Dr Johanna Budwig's book "Flax Oil as a True Aid Against Arthritis, Heart Infarction, Cancer and Other Diseases.")*

Daylight

Dr Budwig focused upon the importance of daylight to our health. It is not enough to absorb electrons only through food, but it is important that we feed ourselves so that our cells are able to absorb and process the light coming from the sun. The more sickly someone is, the sooner he is "in the house", which can be a catastrophic mistake. Especially when people are already in a very late stage of the illness, they are often not able to eat enough and good advice is then very difficult. In such cases, Dr Budwig advises to concentrate on the following three points:

- ELDI oils as whole body rubbings and if possible as enemas
- Only freshly squeezed juices and distributed as food throughout the day if possible the breakfast muesli in different variants
- Stay outside as much as possible

You will experience me to explain what to do next. I have been able to see in my life how Dr Budwig's theoretical considerations work when put to practice, if indeed, if they are consistently carried out. If you could experience such a case yourself, and how quickly it can be better for a seriously ill person, you can see Dr Budwig's words in a very different light.

But other great researchers had also dealt with the subject of light long before Dr Budwig. For example, the anthroposophist Rudolf Steiner wrote, about 50 years earlier that there is a fundamental being of our material existence of the earth, of which all materiality has come only through condensation. Every matter on earth is condensed light! There is nothing in material existence, which is something else than condensed light in some form. Wherever you go and feel matter, you have condensed light everywhere. Compressed light. Matter is light by its very nature. In as much as a man is a material being, he is woven of light. Rudolf Steiner and Dr Budwig have pointed out in their writings over and over again the importance of light and that we humans are now heliotropes, which need light and use light. But I have nowhere else than with Dr Budwig so clearly and understandably read, WHY this is and above all, how the charging of the life battery works and / or what importance mainly the linolenic acid or electron clouds play. Because it is so important, I would like to repeat here again: The sicklier someone is, the more he should be in the open." (Oil-Protein Diet by Lothar Hirneise)

Visualization - Path to wellness

The visualization is perhaps the most important tool to tap into the power of your imagination to help heal cancer, manage problems or rather achieve anything in your life. Learning to direct and control images in your mind can help you to relax. This may help to

- Relieve stress
- Control some of the symptoms caused by your cancer or cancer treatments
- Boost your immune system to help your body fight off infections and promote healing

Past   Future
_____→

Whatever you see around yourself is just a vision in the beginning, For example the cup of coffee you are holding in your hands or the house in which you live today did not exist in the past. Not very long ago there was a thought in your mind that you want to construct a dream house for living. Then you made construction designs and all sort of workup. Our whole life runs on the rails of time and never turns back. This is our time line.

First of all understand that everything around us is just a thought, energy or a wave. It is significant to understand this. Then only you will believe that energy can be converted in to a matter. Just imagine that a hypnotist puts a coin on your palm and makes you believe that it is hot. You feel burning in your palm. You may even have blisters on your palm. Here the temperature of coin just changed through only.

If you have believed that certain thought can change the condition of your body within seconds. Then why not a good thought can heal your tumor. In many studies Visualization trainer Carl Simomton has proved that cancer patients live twice if they follow visualization technique systematically.

Lothar Hirneise, the student of Dr. Johanna Budwig, respects Carl's research too much except a few points. Simomton teaches his cancer patients to visualize that their white cells are attacking cancer cells and killing them. Lothar is against this school of thought. Because in this situation patient focuses on his tumor. But Lothar says that main problem is something else, tumor problem is secondary. Secondly patient thinks of a war with a cancer cell, while Lothar believes that cancer patient needs balance and harmony rather than thinking of a war.

Lothar has interviewed hundreds of cancer survivors and came to the conclusion that cancer patient avoids direct confrontation with his tumor, but wants to remain busy in dealing with healthy and happy future. Though every patient has different approach, but end is same, creating a happy future. Lothar admits that visualization is the single most important therapy in his so much talked about 3E Program. After all if we will not create a healthy future for us then who else will do.

Please, review your time line again and compare it with thought-matter line. You will notice that both lines travel in the same direction and never turn back. You can never change the direction of any line. So start now and create your own happy future yourself.

Thought   Matter

$\longrightarrow$

Past   Future

$\longrightarrow$

I am going to discuss Lothar's technique in detail, which he learned from Europe's famous Visualization trainers Jack Black from Glasgow. Jack has taught his Mind Store System to 50,000 people in last few years. He is consultant of many celebrities and several companies. Lothar recommends that every cancer patient should attend seminars of Jack Black or Klaus Partl. Klaus Partl is right hand of Lothar Hirneise and teaches visualization at his 3E Center in Germany.

Initially Cancer patient thinks that the most important job is to destroy tumor. If he gets rid of tumor then he can plan to take some holistic treatments e.g. visualization. This is very bad decision. It is very important to follow visualization techniques as a part of your tumor destruction program.

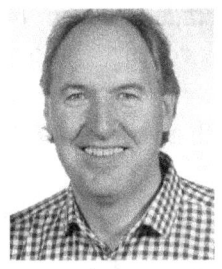

But How does it work? This word HOW is very important, because it usually prevents us to take right decisions. At this moment don't try to think how visualization shall work, how it is going to destroy your tumor. Time being I just say that try to trust us that it actually works.

In short I just say that you learn how to make your future healthy and cheerful, do not focus on present and past. Lothar says that if you know your past, it is easier to change your future. But your main focus should be to create happy future.

Your dream house where you heal your cancer

To give positive impact on your body and mind, it is very important that you become completely relaxed before you start thinking and visualizing. Relaxation or rather achieving alpha stage is the first step. Alpha means relaxed stage (7-14 hertz waves) of your mind. You can relate it with the alpha waves of an EEG tracing. Then there are beta, theta and delta waves. To reach this state there are many techniques or meditations. Some books and CDs are also available. Even listening classical music, meditation or mild yoga can relax you.

When you achieve deep relaxation, start thinking and visualizing. You start it by walking slowly along the right bank of a river. After a short distance you turn towards right. You see blue sky and green meadows. There are lot of trees and a very beautiful house with red terrace. (can imagine your dream house)

Now you enter this house. First room is a beautiful bathroom with a shower. You start taking shower. It washes out all your negativity, toxins and dis-eased cells. After taking shower you sit under the sun, the sunshine dries and fills you with energy within a couple of moments.

Now you go to screen room. On the blank wall of this room there are 3 big LCD monitors. You can relax on the comfortable sofa. You can control these screens with a remote control. On the side table of sofa there also lays a universal DVD recorder. Left screen shows your future, right one the past and the central screen shows your present.

Switch on the central screen, it shows your present sickness. Accept that many people suffered from this illness, you are not alone. Now switch on the right screen to see if you suffered from similar illness in the past. And if you suffered, then how did you treat it. Usually we don't find solution of current problems in the past. Now you minimize and freeze the past screen with remote control. Also, minimize and freeze the present screen.

Now relax and switch on future screen and try to find a solution to your problems. Now visualize a situation where you look perfectly healthy and your tumor has already dissolved. For example if you suffer from bone sarcoma in your thigh and can't even walk due to this illness; you may imagine that you are skiing in Switzerland. Feel the snow peaks, cold breezes, your friend's laughter, your own respiration sounds. Magnify these images, even increase brightness and contrast, and feel the reflection of these images on your body.

You may go to screen room daily, whenever you get time and see yourself skiing. Now you need not to view central and right screen any more. Directly start left screen, our next job is to record this skiing video on universal DVD recorder. The universal DVD recorder will relay this broadcast to the whole world. Your all nears and dears will know about your dream and start helping you to achieve this. To conclude the session, come out of the house and return to the river. Count up to seven and slowly open your eyes. Take a deep breath. This ends your visualization. Always keep in mind that the end should always be happy for everybody; nobody should be harmed any way.

Renovate your dream house if needed

You can construct some extra rooms in this house, if there is a need. For example you can make a small room for rest and relaxation. If you have some pain then you go to this room to relax for a while. You can also make a meeting room. You can invite here some important person to discuss your problem. For example you can call Dr. Johanna Budwig. You can sit with her, discuss and ask her opinion to solve your problem.

You can also invite your friends and close relatives to celebrate your successful skiing expedition. Imagine you are standing on the dice and narrating your experiences and everybody is clapping. The main essence of the story is that in the end people see you are healthy and cheerful. So that they also help you achieve your healthy and happy future. One question is very frequently asked is that how many times you should go to this house. Lothar says that there is no fixed rule but whenever you get time you should visit this house, may be twice a day. If the problem is serious then it is better you go there several times a day.

Visualization wonderfully brings positive changes in your health. It costs nothing but works 100%. You can use this treatment to heal your cancer, make your life happy and cheerful or even to just become a millionaire (Hirneise, 530).

Testimonials

How Dr. Siegfried Ernst cured his stomach cancer

Great healing story written by Dr. Robert Willner

Biography of Dr. Robert Willner

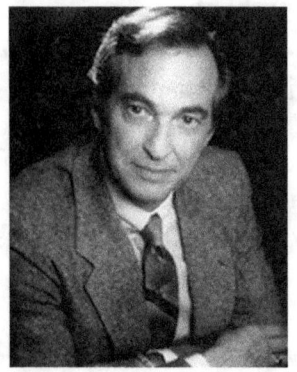

Dr. Robert Willner M.D., PhD (21 June 1929 - 15 April 1995) was an American doctor remembered for his role in AIDS denialism, the view that AIDS is not caused by HIV infection. Willner described himself as originally an "orthodox" physician who slowly changed to alternative medicine, particularly after his wife died of cancer chemotherapy.

In 1995, Willner stated that "I am fully convinced; you can prevent all disease with diet, lifestyle changes and sanitation." Willner wrote some books presenting his point of view on the relation between HIV and AIDS, titled "Deadly Deception: the Proof That Sex And HIV Absolutely Do Not Cause AIDS". The book was published shortly after Wilmer's medical license was revoked for, among other things, treating an AIDS patient with ozone therapy. He also wrote a book about cancer "The Cancer Solutions" after he met Dr. Budwig and studied her protocol in detail.

The following month, on October 28, 1994, in a press conference at a Greensboro, North Carolina hotel, Willner jabbed his finger with blood he said was from an HIV-infected patient. Willner died on April 15, 1995 of heart attack.

Lunch with Dr. Siegfried Ernst

Dr. Robert Willner was very much fascinated by Dr. Johanna Budwig and her cancer research. Dr. Budwig presented clear and scientific evidence, which has been confirmed by hundreds of other related research papers since, that the essential fatty acids were at the core of the answer to the cancer problem. He felt compelled to visit Dr. Budwig in Germany and meet her personally so that he would have the very latest information for his book. So he went to Germany several times before completing his book "The Cancer Solutions."

One day at Dr. Johanna Budwig's residence in Freudenstadt, the phone rang and a happy and lively conversation in German ensued. In a few minutes Dr. Budwig asked him to come to take the phone and said. "This is Dr. Ernst, the friend I told you before. Speak with him and confirm anything you would like."

The conversation with Dr, Ernst lasted approximately ten minutes and Willner tried to remember as much as possible. Most of the facts had already been told to him by Dr. Budwig. Then he returned to the hotel, noted down whatever he could recollect. The next day was Friday and he planned to leave in the morning for Stuttgart. His return flight was on Sunday at eight in the morning. Because it required a very early wake-up and he did not want to any risk. So he decided to arrive there a day early. After purchasing as many of Dr. Budwig's books as possible at a local book shop, he took a taxi to the railway station.

The plane that he had hoped to take was full, and he was advised to get a flight from Munich. On the way to Munich the train stopped at Ulm, which in phone conversation, Dr. Ernst had mentioned was his home. He decided to get off the train and try to meet him. Within an hour he had a room in Golden Tulip Hotel and arranged to meet with Dr. Ernst the next morning. That day there was a lot of fog and snow fall in Ulm and weather was scorching cold. He decided to take sauna bath in health club of the hotel. After sauna bath, he felt warm and fresh. He ordered pucked pride dry wine, avocado vasabi salad and hot sizzling fajita for the dinner.

He spent the next day with Dr. Ernst who seemed very healthy and active, though he was in late seventies. He was famous and dedicated man in the town. He was devoted to family, church, city and humanity. The present Pope and many other dignitaries were his close friends.

Dr. Ernst told that seventeen years ago he developed stomach cancer for which he had major surgery. It had required removal of his stomach and left him with a great number of digestive problems and considerable debilitation. His professional life had practically come to an end. He was approximately sixty years old at the time. He had great difficulty in continuing his clinical practice.

Two years later he had a recurrence of the cancer and was advised chemotherapy as the only available remedy. There was very little hope for survival, and he knew that chemotherapy was not only ineffective, but completely damaging for the quality of life, so he said No to chemotherapy.

Then he went to Dr. Budwig for trying her protocol. For two years he religiously followed the Budwig diet and, also, he used the application of the Flax seed oil to his body every evening. The oil was applied to the abdominal area and wrapped with cloth bandages. He continued the low fat Quark and Flax seed oil daily. It has been fifteen years since the recurrence of the stomach cancer and the institution of the Budwig therapy. Dr. Ernst has had healthy life except some minor problems with eating and digesting food. The simple addition of digestive enzymes and other supplements have made his existence almost completely normal.

Virtually all patients with a recurrence of this type of cancer rarely survive a year, even if they agree to chemotherapy. And the toxic-effects from the chemotherapy makes life more regrettable. Of course the conventional doctors will dismiss the story of Dr. Ernst as a "spontaneous remission" in spite of the fact that it is unheard of, except when patients go for simple alternative therapies.

Their conversation lasted for many hours and he confirmed much of what Dr. Budwig had told him. He recalled the many stories of patients she had treated. He admitted that whatever skepticism he had about this great therapy, disappeared completely after meeting with Dr. Ernst. He was both a colleague and a fellow cancer victim who had been truly cured, not just a five-year survival (Dr Robert E. Willner M.D., 1993, Chapter 5).

Highly positive and encouraging story of Mary

Diagnosis of Cancer and the triple bladed sword: surgery, chemo and radio

I was diagnosed with breast cancer in July 2001. I had two surgeries, 47 sessions of radiation and 4 months of chemo.

Then in June 2005, I was told that the cancer had spread to my spine. I underwent a very extensive surgery on June 11, 2005. The doctor told me that cancer was eating my spine and making it weak and hollow. **They said I have 20 months to live.** They explained me that when cancer spreads to your spine; after a few months for it to spread to other organs such as kidneys, bladder, lungs, etc. Then you die. **But first, they wanted give me radiation and chemo again and again until I die.** So in July 2005, I had only 10 sessions of radiation. After this I was totally exhausted and drained. Then I finally decided NO RADIO! NO CHEMO! Nothing! If I am ready to die, I want to enjoy my death!

Starting on my path to healing

No No No ... how could I die so soon! **I would win this war against breast cancer.** So I jumped into the river Google and came out with bunch of research done by a doctor from Germany in my hand. She had developed a simple cure for cancer. Take cold-pressed organic Flax seed oil with Cottage Cheeseand eat only fresh foods, such as veggies and fruits, and get sunlight.

Terminal breast cancer cured in record time

So I had been taking this natural treatment for 8 months? I had my repeat bone scan, MRI and CT in November. **Not only my cancer vanished, but there is new bone growing in the holes where the cancer ate it away!!!** My oncologist is shocked to see the scans! I am thrilled ☺

Winning my cancer war with a bonus:

This time not only have I won the war against cancer, and let's face it... chemo does not CURE cancer. Flax seed oil combined with sulfurated protein is the ONLY CURE for cancer in my experience. I had a scar tissue in my right breast was about the size of a golf ball, shown up on all my mammograms since my surgery in 2001. It was also there in March 2005 as usual. But in the November mammogram, the scar tissue had reduced to the size of a small coin! I fully expect it to be vanished by the mammogram in March 2006! And apart from this healing, I have lost 70 lbs weight! Just from eating right and exercising! Wow! And I look forward to lose another 10 pounds in July. ☺

Breast Cancer - Miracle healing

Mrs. Neelam 60 yrs. from Almoda suffers from Breast Cancer. She came to me in last Dec. She has not taken any Chemo, Radio or Surgery. I advised her to take Budwig Protocol sincerely. She immediately started the Protocol along with Pranayam, Coffee Enema, Soda bicarb bath and Flax oil massage. She called me yesterday on May 1 and told that her tumor has shrieked more than 50%. This is really a miracle of Budwig Protocol.

Wellness Journey of Mrs. Shanti

This patient Mrs. Shanti 40 years in age belongs to a village near Dungargarh. She came to us in August, 2014 for the first time. She suffered from Leomyosarcoma Uterus (Cancer of Uterus) before one and half years. She was operated and treated by conventional treatment at Bikaner. She remained in remission for six months. After that she developed Metastasis Tumor in Left 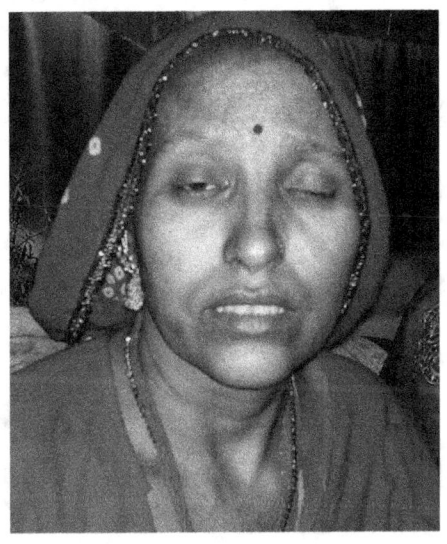 Lumbar region. She also had severe anemia (Hb was 5.7 gm in June, 2014), pain, weakness, ascites, anorexia and vomiting. No treatment was helping her. Then somebody told her to consult me. When I examined her she looked very weak, pale, apathic and drowsy, she hardly spoke anything. Her Hemoglobin was approx. 7 Gm. She had unbearable pain in her left Lumbar region.

The whole family was uneducated and lived in farm in rural area. They do not understand Hindi. It was really very difficult for us to train them, as communication was a big problem. But our audio-visual approach helped and conducted the training anyhow. I was very sure that they will hardly follow Budwig Protocol more than a few days. But after a month and half her brother spoke to me and told that patient is improving slowly and asked some questions. It was a bit strange for me but still I had no hope.

On November 25, 2014 when she stepped in to my clinic, I was totally shocked to see her. What a change! What a miracle!! She was entirely a new woman. She looked active, healthy, happy and young. She was smiling, her face was glowing. Her vomiting stopped, appetite improved and pain reduced. She was talking and asking questions in her local language. She followed the Budwig treatment nicely, and she has not taken any conventional treatment during last four months. This time her Hemoglobin was 11.5 Gm, though we did not prescribe her any iron capsule. Her Metastatic tumor which was 84x78x55 mm in June 10, 2014 has reduced to 46x34 mm, a drastic reduction in size. Liver size became normal and kidney stone passed out. This is a magic of Budwig Protocol. This wellness was achieved by use of Flax oil, the sun shine in a bottle or rather the essence of our life.

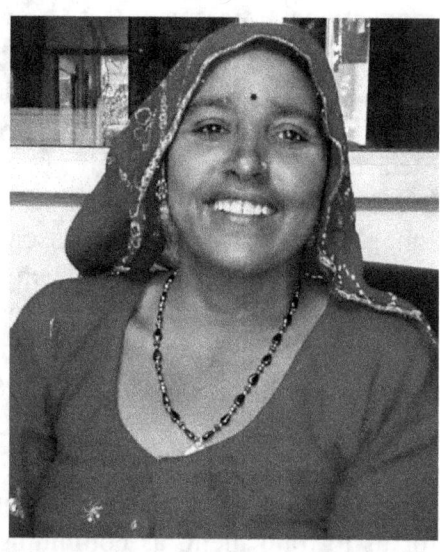

Many people think that Budwig Protocol is just a mixture of Flax oil and cottage cheese. It is biggest mistake one can ever do. Because in real terms Budwig Protocol is much more than that. It is healing of body, mind and spirit. Here the difference between winning and losing is so small that your minute neglect can tip the balance of the whole treatment. And that is why thorough and expert training is so important for every patient who wishes to take Budwig Protocol.

Tom's cured his Brain Cancer

My name is Kelly and on February 10, 2002 I brought my husband to the Emergency with a splitting headache and severe vomiting. We thought it was a migraine attack but later found out that it was a brain tumor. On February 12, he had surgery and the biopsy was done. After lab workup surgeon finally declared that he suffered from Glioblastoma Multiforme Grade 4.

The surgeon called me in his office and told me that he removed the tumor as much as he could and Tom had about 6 months to live if he didn't take radiotherapy. If he took radiation it might give him a year. It was a big shock for me. Tom was 37 years old at that time, so young so loving. I did not lose my sweet husband. We were unable to decide what to do, as a last hope we went for radiation. About a week of radiation and he felt terrible and lost all of his energy.

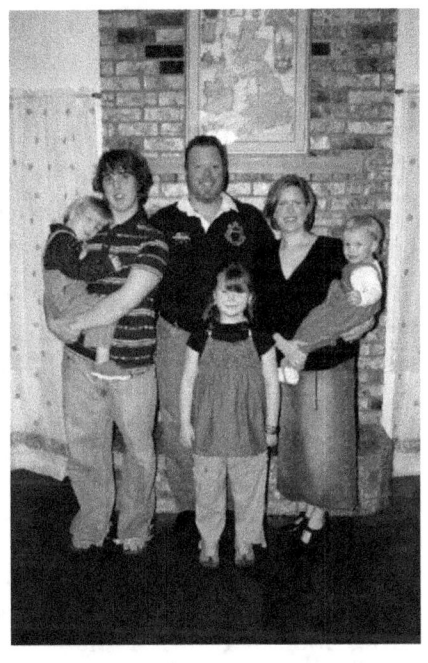

We being Christians, went to church for a prayer. Some friends told us of some alternative therapies. People were fighting and winning the battle against cancer. Dr. Johanna Budwig has had and is having success treating cancer patients with her simple protocol. This way we decided to follow this holistic approach which centered on Flax oil and Cottage Cheesein March.

Tom's three month MRI looked good, his brain scan was clean and the hole where they removed the tumor was empty except for a tiny line around a portion of the inside of the hole. The doctor told that it could be a scar tissue, a benign tumor or a regrowth of the Glioblastoma.

But soon Tom started to recover, began walking for mild exercise and to get some sunlight. We strictly followed the rules and do not eat any pork or fish. It makes it harder for your body to fight cancer if you put unclean and artificial things into it. I think artificial sweetener caused Tom's cancer. He used to drink about 2 liters a day of diet soda every day.

At the six month MRI his brain was completely clean. There was no cancer anywhere. The doctor said that it was a big miracle. In 14 years of practice he had not seen such a healing (CureZone.com).

After 9 months MRI was done in December 2002. He is all right, no sign of any cancer. He started his job and life was back to normal. Praise the Lord Jesus! Dr. Budwig! I am flying in the sky. ☺

Kelly

Healing Story of Jorg Hulf, Hamburg

In September 1980, Jorg Hulf was diagnosed with an adenoid, cystic carcinoma of the tear duct in the left orbital area. He was operated and left eyeball was removed in September 1982. Soon there was a relapse. Again the surgery was performed in the department of oral and maxillofacial surgery in the Oschsenzoll hospital. Doctors told him that his cancer may grow and spread to another eye. So he decided to take the treatment from Dr. Johanna Budwig. Her treatment was scientifically proved, published in medical journals, and is presented at congresses in Germany and abroad (Budwig).

He got the following benefits from using the oil-protein diet and the Eldi oils.

- After surgery the wound healed in a surprisingly short time.
- He had loss of hair in the forehead area, after the first operation. Now hair has grown back in this area.
- He had tooth infection which caused lot of pain, also healed in a short period without ant dental care.
- Blood pressure became normal in a short time and is currently optimal.

140

- Vision of another eye was improved, from 5.8 previously to the present 4.6.
- He was able to do his job after a short time. He felt very good in body and in mind.
- He frequently suffered from migraine headache before the second operation. His migraine attack was very rare and could be managed without medicines.
- Because his family also strictly taking the oil-protein diet, his wife's chronic constipation vegetative dystonia were cured. Previously, she was treated by doctors for years without success. Similar experiences can also be reported for the children.

How Dr. Budwig saved A. Sch

In early 1993 A. Sch noticed a small growth on the right side of her tongue. Because it was irritating her, she had it surgically removed in the E.N.T. Hospital. Same evening her tongue was swollen and became almost black. She had severe pain and had to be admitted in the hospital for three days. But the doctor assured her that the growth was completely harmless.

After about a week, the hospital told her that she had salivary gland cancer. The growth had already spread in the tongue. A new big operation was suggested under general anesthesia. But she refused to sacrifice her tongue and came back home totally shocked. ☹

She called Dr. Budwig, and took a date for an appointment in the coming week. After meeting Dr. Budwig, she was very much satisfied and cheerful. Meanwhile her family doctor called her to his clinic for a discussion. She went to him. He brutally explained her in harsh words that only removal of 3/4 of the tongue could save her life. She refused for the operation politely. After listening this, he forgot the good manners and he became abusive. He said that she would never survive if she did not go for an

141

operation immediately. She said no, to which he 'shouted: OK then go to hell, no body can help you now. During this entire conversation he did not speak a single word of sympathy. She was completely exhausted and hocked. Every hope of healing was gone. This doctor practically pulled the rug out from under her feet. Totally crushed her husband took her to Dr. Budwig. She wiped her tears and gave her new hope through her special and unique manner and spirit.

The very next day, she started the oil-protein diet explained thoroughly by Dr. Budwig. She used to talk her whenever she needed a support. But threats calls from her family doctor kept coming and soon she became mentally very depressed and sad. She had terrible nightmares. Her husband was hardly able to console her after such nightmares. In the dream she always died under the worst situations she could imagine. Soon she lost interest in everything. This doctor had simply sentenced her to death.

After two years of encouragement and sympathetic touch on the part of Dr. Budwig, the nightmares became less frequent and the fear and anxiety slowly vanished completely. She survived the sickness, thanks to Dr. Budwig. Today she was again a happy and healthy person. The oil-protein diet had done wonderful recovery to her. She was very happy that God sent her to Dr. Budwig. How troublesome a life without a tongue would have been, even if she had survived at all. May God bless Dr. Budwig, the great woman (Budwig).

~~**~~

Testimonials on our Budwig Protocol group on FB

Ray Schneider

Well I started Budwig FO/CC on September 25, 2016 and the improvement was noted (CT scans) about three months ago so about March. The interval there is six months, but the timing is in part due to the interval between CT scans. I think I'm continuing to improve but I conclude that only because of reduction is pain experience when coughing or sneezing which used to be sharp and excruciating but has now so decline that at most it is only a slight discomfort and seems to be continuing to decline.

Suzanne Johnson

My husband was diagnosed with prostate cancer, so we started the protocol and 3 months later his PSA had dropped to the point that the doctor said you don't have cancer anymore. Still following protocol will have another test in August to see how he is going, but we think it has gone and we are really enjoying the breakfast and lunch mix and eating vegetarian at night. All the best with your cancer

Kathy Maloney Ormsby

My mom (this is her Face book, I don't have one) did Budwig along with her conventional medicine (surgery where they could, chemo and radiation) when she was diagnosed with Adenocarcinoma NSCLC with brain mets. She only did it for a few months and often cheated on the diet part but was consistent with the FOCC. Since then the cancer has been stable until a few weeks ago we learned a tumor might be forming where she had surgery before so she's doing the FOCC mixture about 2-3 times a day and that's almost all she eats because she's not that hungry. The first time around she was on a heavy dose of steroids to help with the swelling in her brain, this made her very hungry. Today

143

the FOCC is enough to be considered a meal. She also eats apricot kernels, randomly and takes at least 200mg of Laetrile a day. Every situation is different but if I had cancer I would stick to the Budwig Protocol 100% along with Apricot kernels. Six years of taking my mom to oncology appointments changed the way I see medicine. I am confused by the way chronic diseases are approached and treated. Well meaning doctors throw Hail Mary's hoping that their prescriptions or surgery will do the trick without any idea or concern about what the patients are eating. And when we asked the DIETITIAN at the oncology clinic she said she had never heard of Budwig or any of the alternative cures we discussed and recommended she stick to the food pyramid and drink Ensure if not hungry.

Lynn Martinez-Mulimbayan

My tumor marker went down about 4 months after I started my Budwig Diet. But I'm doing fruit-vegetable juicing, coffee enema and taking a bunch of supplements as well. At the end of the year, I was able to confirm I was in remission when I had my PET CT scan.

Allie Hayes

I cured my female Siberian Husky 8 and a half years ago of autoimmune disease with the Cottage CheeseBudwig protocol . She was given approx 1 month to live at age 4 , she lived another 6 yrs and only died sadly of unrelated kidney disease (caused by steroids as she got asthma after her autoimmune disease) .Also my sons very close 25 yr old friend took the diet seriously and followed it strictly when he was given six weeks to live with secondary cancers that had spread into his bones . He lived another 7 months on the diet . Doctors were shocked how long he went on for ! It's well worth trying this diet , helps so many things / ailments not just cancers ! Arthritis is another ailment I have seen 95 % proven improvement of in two people !

Ray Schneider

I've been on the Budwig Protocol since about late September last year and had substantial tumor reduction and it didn't hurt. You do have occasional diarrhea as the body gets rid of the waste and you might want to include some detox methods which Johanna Budwig talks about as well. I personally didn't use any detox methods. I read about them in a variety of books, don't remember which particularly. Coffee enemas was one of the most commonly referenced and I think there were a number of others.

Barry Williams

I have been on the Budwig for 12 months, and my Tumor has shrunk 50% and I am feeling fine. I am 75 and still do all the work around the section.

Niti Shah, U.S.A.

Thank you, Dr. Om Verma !! Love your book and the wealth of information you have put it in there so practically! We are going to follow it and live by it thoroughly.... Also deeply appreciate you being so approachable and responsive to the questions we have! It is not always the case. It is almost impossible to find an ethical doctor these days. I think we found one in you! Keep up the good work and sharing your knowledge with all of us.... I also connected with one of your patient who had a complete recovery from a stage 4 cancer and amazed to hear the patient side of the healing journey! Blessings and best of health.

My Cancer journey with Dr O P Verma and his great book

Hello, my name is Dawne and I live in United States. I am here to share you my cancer experience with Dr Verma's book "Cancer Cause And Cure". It really helped me along my journey. The first three months after I got my diagnosis I was all over the place, I was reading books, I was listening to videos, and I was searching TV, anything and everything that has to do with cancer. One of the biggest problem that I faced was that I was very lonely, I was very afraid and my Oncologist didn't make things better. She was extremely negative and her only way of saying that she was going to cure me was chemo, radiation and surgery. I am on the other hand did not believe in chemo, radiation and surgery. It may have a place in some people but not in my life. I knew that I have to do this through a more holistic natural way. Every part of my body kept telling me not to do chemo and radiation, that there was another way for me and of course I expressed this to my Oncologist and that was a mistake, because she was very negative, she attacked me verbally, calling me a fool, that I am going to die the worst death ever and it was terrifying, it was very scaring.

Like I said, in the First three months I was doing intense research, research of my life and I did a lot of things to heal my cancer and I took everything whatever told me to do it, I did it. I was that afraid so the good news is I must be doing something right when pray to my creator and I ask please guide me in the way, you know you made me, you know how to fix me and undo all the damage that I did to my body because I know I am the one who caused this cancer.

Yes, I have support of my family. Nobody in my family had cancer that knew what to do. So the support they gave me was whatever I decided they would back me up they wouldn't fight me because it is my life. And even I get love from my family I was so alone I was so afraid. Then finally after I was diagnosed I came across a very important book. Oh my goodness, I wish somebody has given me this book at first. It is besides my Bible my creator's word, I consider this my second Bible. The Second most important book in my life and we all know that doctor who wrote this. This is very important to me, but called "Cancer Cause And Cure" and this book really pulled it all together for me. That's the one book that hit me here right in my heart. If I find anybody in my life or if anybody talks about cancer that's the book I am taking him to. It saved my life. It saved my sanity. It kept me from going crazy, wandering, terrified. It was the book that gave me lot of hope. Like I said I don't believe in chemo and radiation. I was already toxic that's why I had cancer, so why I want to put more toxins in my body. The book gave me a lot of reassurance and guidance and that's what I needed. No other book that I had read and believe me I read a lot of books, no other book was as informative as the Cancer Cause And Cure. One of the things about the book in the beginning that it talks about the topic of cancer and two doctor's works, they explain very simply why we get cancer, why I had got cancer and that's the one thing a lot of western medical doctors here in United States won't talk about it. Don't worry how you got? You got it let's cut it out, lets burn it out. And I was before that and I didn't understand scientific medical journals I am not a doctor. I tried to read those book, they terrified me they put me to sleep and I didn't understand what they were talking about. At least with Dr Verma's book I was able to understand a lot of words written there and at least I can work with that. He speaks about the Budwig, the German doctor and that's why I started in the beginning because my sister and I had talked about it a year ago. It's funny, we talked what would we do if we get cancer and we had talked about the Budwig Protocol and once I got my message from my doctor that I had cancer that's the first thing that came into my head Budwig and I read one of Budwig's book. And it helped me learn about what I am supposed to do, but Dr Verma's book made it just a little bit easier to understand because he explains a lot. I was doing the Budwig but I was not doing it quite right, my timing was off. So his book showed me how I am supposed to do it and I got the timing right and another thing with Dr Verma, I thank you so much for being on Face book because whenever I had questions, I was able to ask him you know specific question there and he was so gracious to answer my questions. You know a lot of things when you start doing the Budwig and don't have correct information, you don't really understand how you are supposed to do it correct. Lot of people don't do sauerkraut juice, lot of people don't do teas and champagne. I started to understand this and I made it part of my protocol. I was doing it at first, but I was not doing it completely right. And lot of other things western medical doctors here tell you that there a sun, sun is bad for you causes cancer. Budwig didn't say that. She said you needed it. You need sun, it is important. And Dr Verma's book reiterated that and lot of other therapies that I didn't know about. Some therapies that I was doing were the enemas and again I was not doing it quite right until I got Dr Verma's book. And it explains me that how and what I had to do and I also learned about soaks thorough his book, bath soaks and how to do it? How long to do it? What you should be putting in your bath tubs? Why it is important to do these bath soaks? Another thing that I learned was about supplements. How important they were? And foods you stay away from meats. I used to be a big meat eater. Not anymore no thank you no no no. I have thrown away meat and I eat raw vegetables, fruits, nuts and seeds. That is the base of my diet and I learned that a lot about the Budwig Protocol and other therapies that the book covers. And about pain therapies, I did not know that you can help with pain certain supplements or certain just regular foods. And by Turmeric, Turmeric did a lot for me, it helped in my detox.

And another thing is not in just cancer but diabetes, I used to be, I am type 2 diabetic. I was always told that I will never stop type 2 diabetes. I used to take insulin I used to take pills. With the diet I am on and the ways that I followed the Cancer Cause And Cure book, I no longer have to take medicines for diabetes and also no longer high cholesterol. So the book is wonderful as far as helping me in cancer but helping me in other issues. I also learned to do the mental exercises that the book covers and physical exercises . I am very limited in my abilities to do certain exercises. I walk with the cane. I have my back many years ago. But the exercises they talk in the book taught me how to do things to help my cancer, how to get lymph nodes cleared, how to get lymph system moving and also meditation, I

148

never meditated in my life. And I realize the importance of meditation because he wrote in his book. Also organ cleanses liver cleanses, kidney cleanse and even parasite cleanse. I never thought to do parasite cleanse until I got hold of Dr. Verma's book.

I am glad that he also introduced Lothar Hirneise I read in the book how he was successful in healing patients and that he actually knew Dr Budwig that was so important for me. One of the thing that Lothar covers is the Tumor, how here in United State they will cut the tumor out. And of the thing he specifically says don't do that. Tumor is very important and all along before I even read that I was taught the tumor is just not the cancer, not just the cancer itself, there was more to it, I thought like the tumor was there for important reason, I just don't understand why? But Dr Lothar did and that was good enough for me. And there were many other therapies that other doctors talk about in the book specially dealing with emotions. How emotions help with your past experience and also dealing with people in your life, people that are positive and good for you, but also getting rid of negative people. The first person I got negative was my oncologist. After 3 visits, even when my tumor was shrinking she kept saying you are going die, you are going to die, you have to do this, you have to do chemo, and you have to do radiation. I finally said enough is enough. And I just got off with her. I had another oncologist who is open minded enough. When I told him about what I was doing with the Cancer Cause And Cure and I found Internal Medicine doctor who is integrative, he believes in holistic healing.

One of the thing about The Cancer Cause And Cure book is that you gain an immediate understanding what you got to do. And after first three months I was but once I got the book I followed exactly what it said . I noticed a big difference. First of all I was so calm, I was so relaxed and I put a lot of faith into the book. I now I put my faith in the right ways. This book, you know teaches you how to make the time your friend and the first three months time was not my friend. I thought time was against me. With the book I got to use my time wisely. I don't waste any more time on research. Once I got the Cancer Cause And Cure book that was the end of my research. I knew that I did the right thing by getting the book. And like I said I don't believe Cancer Cause And Cure book is not just for the people with cancer, it's for many other reasons, I feel so much healthier, so much happier.

So Dr Verma from the bottom of my heart, to the top of my heart and throw out my heart, I thank you, I thank you so much for saving my sanity saving my life because the tests that are coming back keep saying that everything is good Sine May and November and I had two tests in between my blood is still clean there is no tumor and there are no swollen nodes and I thank you thank you for being there thank you for writing the book so with that I say farewell you take care and people listen to the book it will save your life Thank you and bless you. Take care...

Mrs Dawne Ulvano U S A

Lucie Bois cured her Breast Cancer by Budwig

I shrunk à big tumor (8.5 cm) in my right breast using Essiac and Budwig protocol. plus lots of fresh homemade veggies juices, organic products, coffee enemas and much more. You got to be committed to à very healthy lifestyle to heal safely.

The tumor has shrunk and could barely be detected on my last Doppler ultrasound test last September and my tumor markers went back into normal range. It took me 2 years and à half to be there. My only challenge now is cancer metastasized as Paget disease of the nipple. Long journey some would say. It would be too long to explain all the protocols I've used (and still using) just on a text. I could say that I used à quite Big arsenal against cancer. Everything God has provide in His nature and non-toxic scientific methods.   I never took chemotherapy, radiations nor any surgery.

Prayer and my faith in à good God who wants the best for me. When you know that you are loved deeply by Creator of the universe who came on earth in the person of Jesus, it gives me assurance. I am also persuaded that God is very unpleased with the corruption in the actual medical system and is raising à squad of uncorrupt Ph.D. and survivors who Will show à different way to heal while respecting the Law of Nature. Now I have a very good reason to heal. It is à mission.

Lucie Bois
Dec 15, 2016

Alisha D'Mello cured her mom's uterine cancer

Hello Dr Verma, thank you for your inspiration and guidance. My mother who has uterine cancer has started the budwig protocol. She is using 2% organic Cottage Cheeseas this is what is available to us. Thank you in advance. Alisha

Posted on Jan 26, 2016

Hello everyone. Wanted to give an update on mom and share some positivity. She was diagnosed with uterine cancer one year ago..with liver met. Chemo was offered but she declined. Started juicing, doing the budwig protocol, cut out meat dairy and sugar, coffee enemas, light exercise and prayer. Liver met was stable after 3 months, started shrinking after another 3 months. She got results for her CT scan today (its been 6 months since the last one) and all clear! She will continue with her diet indefinitely.

Alisha D'Mello
Posted on Dec 17, 2016
(https://www.facebook.com/groups/budwig)

Georgetta

April 9, 2008 – Multiple Myeloma – Georgetta wrote: …my husband has Multiple Myeloma…a very aggressive cancer. He is doing very well on Budwig protocol, lived already beyond Dr's expectation. However, he is not doing chemo. He had a stem cell

151

transplant in 2005, but that did not put him in remission. He started Budwig protocol in 2006, and since then he's been doing only that.
8/16/07-: at Mayo for 3-month visit...tests show no trace of cancer.

History: June 12,'07 – Georgeta wrote: – diagnosed with MM stage III B (Kidney failure) in spring 2005 treated by Mayo doctor with steroids (dexamethasone) for 4 months to restore kidney function. Had stem cell transplant- extremely sick during transplant, almost dead with infections including septicemia. Jan. 2006 while in hospital again, diagnosed with amyloidosis in his lung, another deadly disease. Declared terminal...6 month or less to live -came home extremely sick, unable to eat, sleep, depressed, developed shingles...Found Budwig books on Internet & later FlaxseedOil2 group. Started protocol partially, not being able to eat normal portions. Gradually went on protocol 100%.

Bruce

Sept 2009 - Myeloma - Bruce wrote: "My original diagnosis in January 2007 was IGMK Myeloma...I followed the... Budwig... foods. Within 14 weeks, my counts were dead center normal. 3 months later, my counts were essentially the same. I then stopped my protocol.

Sept 2008, I was rediagnosed with...multiple myeloma with complications that should have caused my death. I refused the allopathic protocol... On 9/17/09, Bruce wrote: I just received my latest blood and urine test results. Other than SLIGHT anemia, all others ARE NORMAL...."

Dheeru Bhai conquered myeloma

Mr. Dheeru Bhai Bohra, aged 89 years, resident of Kandivali, Mumbai, was investigated as pre-operative workup, for the operation of hernia seven years ago. The investigations showed that he has a tumor called plasmacytoma in his stomach.

With the operation of hernia, the lump of their stomach was also removed. Radiotherapy was also given, but after two months, he developed a lump in his shoulder again. The doctors told him that he has now been diagnosed with Multiple Myeloma and chemotherapy should be given. But chemotherapy caused some heart problem, So chemotherapy had to be stopped. Then one of his friends advised to take the treatment of Johanna Budwig. Johanna's treatment led to her recovery. He is completely healthy today and goes to his factory daily. I talked to him before a couple of years. He told me that he is healthy and doing office work in his factory.

~~**~~

The Budwig Diet quotes

"What she (Dr. Johanna Budwig) has demonstrated to my initial disbelief but lately, to my complete satisfaction in my practice is: CANCER IS EASILY CURABLE, the treatment is dietary/lifestyle, the response is immediate; the cancer cell is weak and vulnerable; the precise biochemical breakdown point was identified by her in 1951 and is specifically correctable, in vitro (test-tube) as well as in vivo (real)... "

Dr. Dan C. Roehm M.D. FACP (Oncologist and former cardiologist) in 1990

"Cancer patients suffer from a faulty metabolism caused by a malfunction in the lipid defense system. By repairing the lipid defense system the cancer cannot survive. Of course common chemo and radiation causes further harm to the lipid defense system -- the very system that protects you from cancer! The folks who will READILY ADMIT that they don't understand the cancer mechanism will tell you with their next breath that cancer can be killed with poisons. So can you. Would you trust your car to a so-called mechanic who didn't understand what makes a car work properly? If not, why would you let someone who doesn't understand cancer "fix" your body? The average cancer docs don't know - they admit it. That doesn't make them bad people; it just makes them unqualified to treat your condition if you have cancer. Don't let unqualified people poison you just because they don't know what else to do".

William Kelley Eidem, author "The Doctor Who Cures Cancer (Dr Revici)

"To sell chemotherapy as 'therapy' is most likely the biggest deceit in the history of medicine. Whoever masterminded this chemo-torture deserves a monument in the hell."

Dr. Ryke Geerd Hamer

"I have the answer to cancer, but American doctors won't listen. They come here and observe my methods and are impressed. Then they want to make a special deal so they can take it home and make a lot of money. I won't do it, so I'm blackballed in every country."

Dr Budwig

Dr Rudin believes the Omega 3 story parallels the story of Beriberi & Pellagra. It took them 200 years to accept pellagra was a nutrient deficiency.

"Nobody seemed to notice that a crime has been committed: It was the case of the missing nutrient. The nutrient was essential; it was a nutrient we human beings needed in order to stay healthy. It started to disappear from our diet about 75 years ago and now is almost gone. Only about 20% of the amount needed for human health and well-being remains. The nutrient is a fatty acid so important and so little understood that I call it "the nutritional missing link"....Food grade linseed oil & fish oil are the best sources of this special fat—Omega 3 essential fatty acid—which modern food destroys."

Donaldo Rudin, M.D. (The Omega 3 Phenomenon)

In a 1994 study of 121 women with breast cancer, those in more advanced stages whose breast cancer had spread to their lymph nodes showed the lowest levels of omega-3 fatty acids in the breast tissue. After 31 months, the 20 women who had developed metastases had significantly lower levels of these EFAs (Essential fatty acids) than those who didn't. Another study out of Boston University using the same type of tissue profiles that were used in the breast cancer study demonstrated that patients with coronary artery disease likewise had low levels of EFAs.

"The association between fats—meaning saturated, refined w6s (Omega 6), rancid fats, processed oils, and altered fats---and cancer, (but excluding w3s and fresh, natural, unrefined oils) has long been documented. (They) interfere with oxygen use in our

155

cells. Heat, hydrogenation, light, and oxygen produce chemically altered fat products that are toxic to our cells....These fats kill people. Healing fats in cancer include...... Omega 3s, enhance oxygen use in cells, decrease tumor formation, slow tumor growth, decrease tumor formation, decrease the spread of cancer cells (metastasis), and extend the patient's survival time. Unsaturated fatty acids in fresh, unheated oils are anti-mutagenic. Saturated fatty acids to not have this protective ability. Heating these oils above 150^0 C makes them lose their protective power, and they become mutation-causing. ALL mass market oils except virgin olive oil have undergone heating during deodorization...When we use virgin olive oil or other unrefined oils for sautéing; frying...we overheat them, destroying their protective, anti-mutagenic properties. ALL hydrogenated and partially hydrogenated products have also been overheated.."

Udo Erasmus (Fats That Heal, Fats That Kill)

"Our immune system, which is vital for destroying cancer cells, requires EFAs, vitamins C, B6, and A, and zinc to function, and requires an exceptionally rich nutrient supply of ALL essential nutrients for its high level of complex cellular activities. Deficiencies of EFAs and toxic, man-made synthetic drugs that interfere with essential fatty acid functions can create the conditions of fatty degeneration collectively known as cancer."

Udo Erasmus

"Compared to 100 years ago, Omega 3 is down 80%, B vitamins are estimated to be down to about 50% of the daily requirement. Vitamin B6 consumption may be low as it is removed in grain milling and not replaced. Vitamins B1, B2, B3 and E have also been lost in food processing. Minerals are depleted in a similar way. Fiber is down 75-80%. Ant nutrients have increased substantially---saturated fat, 100%; cholesterol, 50%; refined sugar nearly 1000%; salt up to 500%; and funny fat isomers nearly 1,000%."

Dr Rudin

Dr. Johanna Budwig is rightly known far beyond the borders of Germany. Her ingenious, simple, and effective oil-protein diet has found adherents throughout the world and it has helped many people to particularly better deal with their cancer illness.

I had the great good fortune of spending many days in discussion with her over a period of several years, of being able to study her extensive case histories, of giving joint presentations with her, and of thus gaining an understanding of nutrition for myself that extended far beyond that which I was previously able to find in the usual literature. But what was most convincing to me in my activity on the executive board of Menschen gegen Krebs in Germany was the oil-protein diet.

Hardly a day goes by when I do not talk with people on the phone that has changed their diet along the guidelines provided by Dr. Budwig. I am party first-hand to how successful this nutrition therapy is. I consciously use the term nutrition therapy and not cancer diet because I think it would be an injustice to Dr. Budwig to not to distinguish her scientifically grounded oil-protein therapy from all the diets that are offered around the world.

For me the oil-protein diet always serves as the basis of a cancer therapy and please understands that I am not just simply writing this, but that I have carefully chosen my words, as I have become familiar with more than 100 different alternative cancer therapies in recent years, and I have investigated many of them. When Dr. Johanna Budwig died the cancer scene lost one of the last great scientists of the last century, and it behooves each of us to carry her legacy to future generations, so that they as well can profit from the oil-protein diet.

Lothar Hirneise

I am referring to a super nutrient, which has been neglected for decades, it is neither taught properly in the schools, nor the doctors discuss about it openly, multinationals have removed this from our diet, but the hard truth is that it is essential for our body, it keeps us healthy and fit, protects us from many serious ailments, its presence is essential for cellular respiration, our cells suffocate in its absence, without this our life is impossible, name of this nutrient is alpha-linolenic acid, which is head of the omega-3 family and the richest food source is FLAX SEED OIL.

Dr. O.P. Verma, Flax Guru

They (American Cancer Society) lie like scoundrels.

M. Dean Burk PhD who worked for the National Cancer Institute for 34 years

There have been many cancer cures, and all have been ruthlessly and systematically suppressed with a Gestapo-like thoroughness by the cancer establishment.

Robert C. Atkins MD

Essiac Is A Cure For Cancer. I've seen it reverse and eliminate cancers at such a progressed state that nothing medical science currently has could have accomplished similar results. I wouldn't have believed it myself had I not seen it with my own eyes. I feel very strongly that Essiac is the single most beneficial treatment for cancer today.

C.A. Brusch, M.D., J.F.K's personal physician talking to radio talk show host and producer Elaine Alexander in a radio broadcast from Vancouver, British Columbia, in November 1984

The War Against Quackery is a carefully orchestrated, heavily endowed campaign sponsored by extremists holding positions of power in the orthodox hierarchy.....The multimillion-dollar campaign against quackery was never meant to root out incompetent doctors; it was, and is, designed specifically to destroy alternative medicine...The millions were raised and spent because orthodox medicine sees alternative, drugless medicine as a real threat to its economic power. And right they are...the majority of the drug houses will not survive.

Dr Atkins, M.D. (The Healing of Cancer by Barry Lynes)

And what do I actually do? I give cancer patients simple, natural foods. That is all. I take sick people out of the hospital, when it is said there that they do not have more than an hour or two left to live, that the scientifically attested diagnosis is at hand and that the patient is completely moribund. In most cases I can help even these patients quickly and conclusively.

Dr. Johanna Budwig, in "Flax Oil as a True Aid"

Cancer has only one prime cause. It is the replacement of normal oxygen respiration of the body's cells by an anaerobic (i.e., oxygen-deficient) cell respiration.

Dr. Otto Warburg, twice Nobel Laureate

...the cause of cancer is no longer a mystery; we know it occurs whenever any cell is denied 60% of its oxygen requirements.

Cancer, above all other diseases, has countless secondary causes. But, even for cancer, there is only one prime cause. Summarized in a few words, the prime cause of cancer is the replacement of the respiration of oxygen in normal body cells by a fermentation of sugar. All normal body cells meet their energy needs by respiration of oxygen, whereas cancer cells meet their energy needs in great part by fermentation. All normal body cells are thus obligate aerobes, whereas all cancer cells are partial anaerobes.

Dr. Otto Warburg Prime Cause and Prevention of Cancer

[C]hemotherapy is basically ineffective in the vast majority of cases in which it is given.

Ralph Moss, PhD, former Director of Information for Sloan Kettering Cancer Research Center

159

Three Australian oncologists - Associate Professor Graeme Morgan, Professor Robyn Ward and Dr. Michael Barton - undertook a meta-analysis aiming to determine the actual contribution of cytotoxic chemotherapy to survival in adult cancer patients. Their results, published in "Clinical Oncology" in 2004 under the title "The contribution of cytotoxic chemotherapy to 5-year survival in adult malignancies" (abstract available at www.ncbi.nlm.nih.gov/pubmed/15630849) found the overall contribution of these drugs to 5-year survival in adults to be an estimated 2.3% in Australia and 2.1% in the USA. See Table: Impact of cytotoxic chemotherapy on 5-year survival in American adults showing the percentage of 5-year survivors after chemotherapy for 22 types of cancer. The authors concluded that "it is clear that cytotoxic chemotherapy only makes a minor contribution to cancer survival".

A detailed review of this important paper is owed to Dr. Ralph Moss and can be read for instance at www.icnr.com/articles/ischemotherapyeffective.html under the title "How Effective Is Chemo Therapy?"

Healing Cancer Naturally

"Best book I've ever read on chemotherapy."

Ralph Moss' Questioning Chemotherapy is a book that every person faced with cancer must read before submitting to toxic chemicals which may very well destroy the body's immune system. Unlike many alternative health authors who base their conclusions on anecdotal evidence, Moss uses the medical establishment's own research to prove that in almost all instances chemotherapy is NOT a viable approach to improving cancer survival rates. Moss also makes the important point that current cancer research has never bothered to examine the mental anguish, physical suffering, and poor quality of life endured by almost everyone whose doctors talk or scare them into undergoing chemotherapy. Learning about the economics behind chemotherapy drives the final nail into the coffin of a "therapy" that educated people in the future will consider outrageous and reflective of the current dark ages of so-called modern medicine. This is a must read book for anyone who wants to know the truth behind chemotherapy or anyone whose doctor wants to inject toxic chemicals into their bloodstream.

Chet Day's review of "Questioning Chemotherapy: A Critique of the Use of Toxic Drugs in the Treatment of Cancer" by Ralph W. Moss

Except for two forms of cancer, chemotherapy does not cure. It tortures and may shorten life...

Dr. Candace Pert, Georgetown University

Chemo drugs are some of the most toxic substances ever designed to go into a human body, their effects are very serious, and are often the direct cause of death. Like the case of Jackie Onassis, who underwent chemo for one of the rare diseases in which it generally has some beneficial results: non-Hodgkin's lymphoma. She went into the hospital on Friday and was dead by Tuesday.

Dr Tim O'Shea in TO THE CANCER PATIENT

Cancer researchers, medical journals, and the popular media all have contributed to a situation in which many people with common malignancies are being treated with drugs not known to be effective.

Dr. Martin Shapiro UCLA

~~**~~

Disclaimer

This book is not intended to replace the advice and/or care of a qualified health care professional. Please do not try to self diagnose or self treat any disease. Seek professional help and consult your physician before making any dietary changes.

This book is not intended to provide medical advice and is sold with the understanding that the publisher and the author have neither liability nor responsibility to any person or entity with respect to loss, damage or injury caused or alleged to be caused directly or indirectly by the information contained in this book or the use of any products mentioned. Readers should not use any of the product discussed in this book without the advice of a medical profession.

The Food and Drug Administration has not approved the use of any of the natural treatments discussed in this book. This book, and the information contained herein, has not been approved by the Food and the Drug Administration.

My Book

Cancer - Cause and Cure
Based on Quantum Physics developed by Dr. Johanna Budwig

http://www.amazon.com/Cancer-Quantum-Physics-developed-Johanna-ebook/dp/B00P3Y7BYG

Book Description

***** A must have book for every cancer patient *****

This book provides an introduction of Dr. Budwig's cancer research and treatment. Johanna

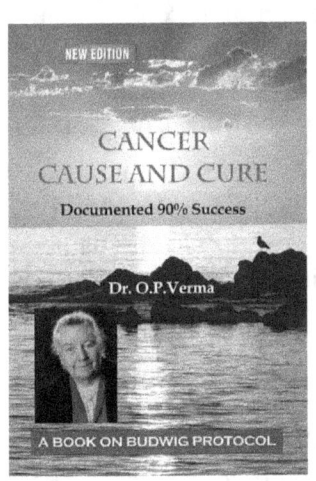

Budwig (1908-2003) was nominated for the Nobel Prize seven times. She was one of Germany's leading scientists of the 20th Century, a biochemist and cancer specialist with a special interest in essential fats.

Otto Warburg proved that prime cause of cancer oxygen-deficiency in the cells. In absence of oxygen cells ferment glucose to produce energy, lactic acid is formed as a byproduct of fermentation. He postulated that sulfur containing protein and some unknown fat is required to attract oxygen in the cell.

In 1951 Dr. Budwig developed Paper Chromatography to identify fats. With this technique she proved that electron rich highly unsaturated Linoleic and Linolenic fatty acids were the undiscovered mysterious decisive fats in respiratory enzyme function that Otto Warburg had been unable to find. She studied the electromagnetic function of pi-electrons of the linolenic acid in the membranes of the microstructure of protoplasm, for all nerve function, secretions, mitosis, as well as cell break-down.

163

This immediately caused lot of excitement in the scientific community. New doors could open in Cancer research. Hydrogenated fats, including all Trans fatty acids were proved as respiratory poisons.

Then Budwig decided to have human trials and gave flaxseed oil and quark to cancer patients. After three months, the patients began to improve in health and strength, the yellow green substance in their blood began to disappear, tumors gradually receded and at the same time the nutrients began to rise. This way Dr. Budwig had found a cure for cancer. It was a great victory and first milestone in the battle against cancer. Her treatment protocol is based on the consumption of flax seed oil with low fat cottage cheese, raw organic diet, mild exercise, and the healing powers of the sun. She treated approx. 2500 cancer patients during a 50 year period with this protocol till her death with over 90% documented success.

She was nominated 7 times for Nobel Prize but with a condition that she will use chemotherapy and radiotherapy with her protocol. They did not want to collapse the 200 billion dollar business over night. She always refused to support the damaging chemo and radio for the sake of humanity.

Lothar Hirneise is founder and President of People Against Cancer, Germany. He travels a lot in search of finding most successful alternative cancer therapies. He has been student of Dr. Johanna Budwig. He is a great researcher and writer on alternative healing. He is successfully treating thousands of cancer patients at his 3-E center in Germany. In the last few years he has interviewed several hundred final stage so-called survivors, meaning patients who were in the final stage of cancer and who are all healthy again today. Based on his findings he proposed a 3 E Program – The Mnemonic of Cancer Treatment.

1) Eat well

2) Eliminate

3) Energy

He noticed that 100% of all survivors, did the energy work. In approximately - say 80% of all patients, had changed their diet. And in at least 60% of all patients, took intensive detoxification rituals. This is the basis of his, so much talked about 3E Program for healing cancer.

Lothar Hirneise strongly supports holistic and spiritual approach and includes Visualization, Tumor Contract, Meditation, mild Yoga, Emotional Freedom Technique, Dr. Ryke Geerd Hamer's New German Medicine (Connection of unresolved stress and cancer), Detoxification techniques (Soda Bicarb bath, Epsom bath, Sauna, Colon Hydrotherapy, Coffee Enema etc.) in his 3 E Program.

The book also, describes about rare and miraculous herbs used in the treatment of Cancer like Turmeric, Black seed, Ginger, Mistle Toe, Aloe vera, Echinecea, Lobelia, Essiac Tea, Pau d'arco Tea, Dandelion, Milk Thistle.

~~**~~

Awesome Flax: A Book by Flax Guru

http://www.amazon.com/Awesome-Flax-Book-Guru-ebook/dp/B00PUUIR0K

Flax seed- Miraculous Anti-ageing Divine Food

What is Flax seed and how can it benefit me? I was faced with this question when I started hearing about Flax seed not long ago. It became a 'buzz word' in society and seems to be making great role in increased health for many. I wanted to join that wagon of wellness and so I researched until I felt satisfied that it could help me, too. Here are my findings.

Flax seeds are the hard, tiny seeds of Linum usitatissimum, the Flax plant, which has been widely used for thousands of years as a source of food and clothing. Flax seeds have become very popular recently, because they are a richest source of the Omega 3 essential fatty acid; also known as Alpha Linolenic Acid (ALA) and lignans. People in the new millennium may see Flax seed as an important new FOOD SUPER STAR. In fact, there's nobody who won't benefit by adding Flax seed to his or her diet. Even Gandhi wrote: "Wherever Flax seed becomes a regular food item among the people, there will be better health."

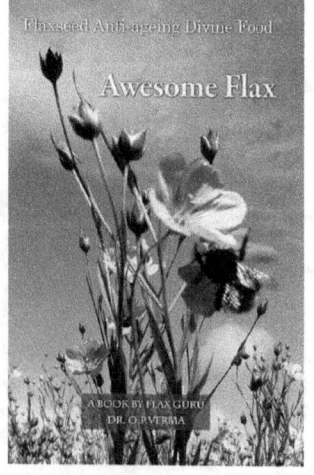

Flax seed contains 30-40% oil (including 36-50% alpha linolenic acid, 23-24% linoleic acid- Omega-6 fatty acids and oleic acids), mucilage (6%), protein (25%), Vitamin B group, lecithin, selenium, calcium, folate, magnesium, zinc, iron, carotene, sulfur, potassium, phosphorous, manganese, silicon, copper, nickel, molybdenum, chromium, and cobalt, vitamins A and E and all essential amino acids.

166

Other fatty acids, omega-6's, is abundant in vegetable oils such as corn, soybean, safflower, and sunflower oils as well as in the many processed foods made from these oils. Omega-6 fatty acids have stimulating, irritating and inflammatory effect while omega-3 fatty acids have calming and soothing effect on our body. Our bodies function best when our diets contain a well-balanced ratio of these fatty acids, meaning 1:1 to 4:1 of omega-6 and omega-3. But we typically eat 10 to 30 times more omega-6's than omega-3's, which is a prescription for trouble. This imbalance puts us at greater risk for a number of serious illnesses, including heart disease, cancer, stroke, and arthritis. As the most abundant plant source of omega-3 fatty acids, Flax seed helps restore balance and lets omega-3's do what they're best at: balancing the immune system, decreasing inflammation, and lowering some of the risk factors for heart disease.

One way that Omega 3 essential fatty acid known as Alpha Linolenic Acid ALA helps the heart is by decreasing the ability of platelets to clump together. Flax seed helps to lower high blood pressure, clears clogged coronaries, lowers high blood cholesterol, bad LDL cholesterol and triglyceride levels and raises good HDL cholesterol. It can relieve the symptoms of Diabetes Mellitus. It lowers blood sugar level. Flax seed help fight obesity. Adding Flax seed to foods creates a feeling of satiation. Furthermore, Flax seed stokes the metabolic processes in our cells. Much like a furnace, once stoked, the cells generate more heat and burn calories.

Flax seeds are the most abundant source of lignans. Lignans are plant-based compounds that can block estrogen activity in cells, reducing the risk of Breast, Uterus, Colon and Prostate cancers. According to the US Department of Agriculture, Flax seed contains 27 identifiable cancer preventative compounds. Lignans in Flax seeds are 200 to 800 times more than any other lignan source. Lignans are phytoestrogens, meaning that they are similar to but weaker than the estrogen that a woman's body produces naturally. Therefore, they may also help alleviate menopausal discomforts such as hot flashes and vaginal dryness. They are also antibacterial, antifungal, and antiviral.

Because they are high in dietary fiber, ground Flax seeds can help ease the passage of stools and thus relieve constipation, hemorrhoids and diverticular disease. Taken for inflammatory bowel disease, Flax seed can help to calm inflammation and repair any intestinal tract damage.

~~**~~

Secrets of Success: Smart way to success for every student

http://www.amazon.com/Secrets-Success-Smart-success-student-ebook/dp/B00Q3IIVAO/

Secrets of Success

Normally people think that memory, intelligence or learning ability is a God gift and it is not possible to further improve or increase the brain powers. We take it for granted that it will remain as it is gifted to us by God. But the truth is just opposite. Understand that as you go to gym for workout to develop your six pack abs, feed your body with muscle building food and get sharp sculpted body shape. Friends, believe me if muscle can be built and remodeled, then why not your brain's hardware and circuit boards. If you feed your brain with proper food it needs, follow simple instructions and take advantage of neurobics or mnemonics, you can immensely increase your brain's abilities.

We have tremendous powers locked inside our brains, but we are not using them to full extent. Dr. William James, considered the father of modern psychology, pointed out that "the average human being uses only 10 percent of his mental capacity." We still have to find out how much power or secrets are hidden in our brain.

Nowadays scientists have discovered mysterious techniques and nutrients to boost our brain powers. Today I shall raise curtains from all these secrets; I shall disclose all hidden tricks and tips. Today you are going to learn how your CPU, the brain tightly packed in a bony cabinet, functions. I teach you how each component and microprocessors works and how the best insulation material can be prepared. I also disclose the right technique to sharpen your brain and to make you an intelligent and successful scholar.

Today you will learn how to crack every examination you face, solve every question, defeat every opponent and get highest possible marks. You are going to write new equation of education and success.

Friends new boundaries and horizon of success is ready to welcome you. Today we shall discuss in detail about some great nutrients and supplements to boost your memory, learning, imagination, creativity and concentration. If you follow our suggestions and apply simple tricks you achieve a successful personality. This short e-book is going to prove a turning point in your life. Wish you luck.

Cancer Cure Is Found: Letrile is the answer

https://www.amazon.com/Cancer-Cure-Found-Laetrile-answer/dp/1797710206/

CANCER CURE IS FOUND

During 1950, a biochemist Dr. Ernest T. Krebs Jr., isolated a new vitamin from bitter apricot kernel that he called 'B-17' or 'Laetrile'. He conducted further lab animal and culture experiments to conclude that laetrile would be effective in the treatment of cancer. He proposed that cancer was caused by a deficiency of Vitamin B 17 (Laetrile, Amygdaline). Laetrile is a concentrated and purified form of vitamin B17. After a lot of research, he had finally developed a specific protocol to treat cancer. Laetrile Therapy combines Laetrile with nutritional supplements and a healthy diet to create a potent treatment that fights cancer cells while helping to strengthen the body's immune system.

Vitamin B-17, which is present in several different foods, consists of a locked substance which comprises two units' glucose, one unit benzaldehyde and one unit cyanide. When B17 comes in contact with a cancer cell it is unlocked by a hormone found only in the cancer cell, and becomes a lethal chemical bomb which destroys the cancer cell. Healthy cells do not cause breakdown of B17. Cancer is unknown to people living in areas with food products rich in B-17, and the population lives to a remarkably high age. Apparently nature has provided us with an ingenious defense against cancer, and it is an ordinary nutrient in our food. These are, amongst others nuts, seeds, vegetables, and in particular apricot kernels.

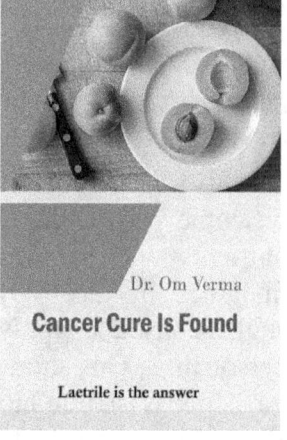

Dr. Om Verma

Cancer Cure Is Found

Laetrile is the answer

At present, patients listen or read a lot about Laetrile treatment, but usually they don't get precise and to the point information about what are the exact components of this protocol, where to get Laetrile injections and supplements, what to take, what not to take, what are the doses, how long to take the treatment, what diet they have to follow, etc. In this book, I have explained the protocol in detail proposed by Dr. Krebs. I have given every minute detail about Laetrile, other nutritional supplements and diet in this book. After reading this book patients can buy Laetrile injections, tablets and other nutritional supplements from the reliable sources (given in the book) and conduct the treatment under the supervision of their family doctor. Dr. Philip E. Binzel was personally trained by Dr. Ernest T. Kreb Jr. about everything of this treatment. Dr. Binzel had been using Laetrile therapy in the treatment of cancer patients since the mid 1970s. His record of success was astounding. Testimonies of his patients are also included in this book.

www.ingramcontent.com/pod-product-compliance
Lightning Source LLC
Chambersburg PA
CBHW051311220526
45468CB00004B/1298